Sick and Tired

Race, Medicine, and Jazz

by
Richard Garcia, MD

Sick and Tired

Race, Medicine, and Jazz

by
Richard Garcia, MD

Foreword

by

Enrique D. Rigsby, Ph.D.

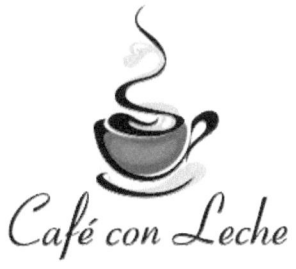

Sick and Tired: Race, Medicine, and Jazz

© Copyright 2020, Richard Garcia, MD

Cover art & design by Miles Garcia

ISBN: 978-1-7328303-2-5

All rights reserved. No part of this publication may be reproduced, stored in a retrieval system, or transmitted in any form or by any means—electronic, mechanical, photo-copy, recording, or any other—except for brief quotations in printed reviews, without the prior written consent of the author.

Published by

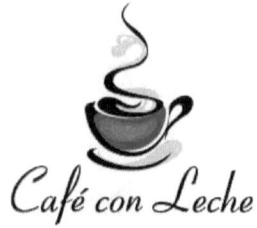

3 Griffin Hill Court
The Woodlands, TX 77382
281-465-0119
www.cafeconlechebooks.com

Dedication

For the Garcia children. And for Vicky.

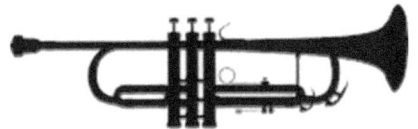

Table of Contents

Foreword ix

Part One Framing Solutions **1**

1 John Henry is Dead 3
2 Poor 15
3 Marble Rye 29
4 Distractions 45
5 Revoltist 65

Part Two Barriers and Old Ideas **79**

6 Dismantling 81
7 Where's Barrington? 95
8 In Baltimore, Once 105
9 Think 117
10 Jesus of Exeter 129

Part Three The Audience and New Ideas **143**

11 Two Instants 145
12 I Can Bleed for Myself 157
13 Seeing Norman Lear 165
14 Bryan Stevenson 177
15 Monk Played in the Cracks 193

"I am sick and tired of being sick and tired."
Tombstone Inscription
Fannie Lou Hamer
Civil Rights Leader

October 6, 1917 – March 14, 1977

Foreword

The insightfully astute reading of Aristotle, William Faulkner, Toni Morrison, and Thelonious Monk has rendered astonishing access into the mind of the undeniable genius that is Richard Garcia. It's an unlikely story, but one you cannot ignore. A medical doctor who rises from the poverty of Stockton, California to become a poet, jazz aficionado, student of literature and arts, published author and captivating speaker, integrates those influences to agitate the status quo regarding American race relations in general, and how race colors the practice of healthcare in particular.

This brilliant work finds its locus at the intersection of music, literature, and medicine, beginning with a clarion call from civil rights legend Fannie Lou Hamer. Sadly, her words are just as in play today as they were six decades ago. On one occasion, the co-founder of the Mississippi Freedom Democratic Party chose nationwide television as the platform to ask a racially divided country, "Is this America . . . the land of the free and the home of the brave?" Hamer's voice echoes today with a piercing familiarity among not only those who exist along the periphery of mainstream society, but to cadres of publics who relentlessly pursue liberation in all forms.

As race shapes the context of health disparities in America, red-herring justifications impinge upon the realities of many and reduce the voices of truth to little more than a distant whimper, plagued by shallow rhetoric and formulaic practice. Former Surgeon General David Satcher, MD, Ph.D. put it quite clearly when he asked in an article, "What If We Were Equal?" A Comparison of The Black-White Mortality Gap In 1960 And 2000." The fact that ethnic populations are dissimilar to others in 2020 represents a blatant incongruence in a society that prides itself on innovation, collaboration, and diversification.

Garcia's assertion, "The rhetorical location remains with the healthcare 'system,' which makes a discussion about our system an unreality," serves as both a general theme and cautionary tale for those in positions to recommend and implement change. More schools that produce more minority doctors obviously is not the answer. Perhaps the question is wrong. Instead of asking how to eradicate disparities, the real question ought to be: *Are we willing to learn a different way from those who have practiced before us?* Different is not defined as inferior.

Foreword

We treat health disparities the way we treat other issues in need of serious debate. We don't. The statement that "we should have improved healthcare for all" is mindlessly nebulous, but it makes us feel good. Trite and overused speak about health disparities is analogous to talking about Black History Month. The scant mention is motivated not by a desire to learn from our history, but because the month appears on our social calendar and appeases our sense of justice and the myth of democracy. Besides, mentioning Black History Month, combined with attending an event in February, may offer the illusion of *overcoming* without marches and sit-ins. In other words, the rhetorical control tactic of *avoidance*, as coined by researchers Bowers and Ochs, can allow one to celebrate the advances of African Americans without addressing systemic inequities (*The Rhetoric of Agitation and Control*, John Bowers and Donovan Ochs, Waveland Press, 1971). Perhaps the custodians of traditional practices may need reminding that disparities don't dissolve in February and that people are Black all year long. In the words of Civil Rights pioneer Reverend Fred Shuttlesworth, "Baseball teams don't strike themselves out. Rattlesnakes don't commit suicide."

As a minister and student of church history, I always have been fascinated by how society members rank-order sin. We'll say, "My sin is not as bad as yours," and so forth.

Our healthcare rhetorical diet seems to rank-order, as well, with choices including exclusivity, entitlement, White, non-White, rich, and poor, all adding layers of bureaucracy to debate, while offering privilege to some, and bondage to others, based on economics and race. What would Jesus say about *that*?

The audience is key in communication. Garcia uses jazz to help audience members think about deeply, and evaluate critically, the interplay between race and medicine. Garcia's chapters "Are not recipes that can be deployed like, say, a recipe for oatmeal cookies." Rather, through systemic changes based on common sense and historical considerations, more authentic dialogue may emerge.

Current medical practices and their supporting literature begs the question, "Who is the intended audience when writing about disparities between races?" At present, *ethos* is missing. Credibility cannot be fabricated from one-sided rhetorical pronouncements. Jazz music instructs us that meaning is derived through the transactional dialogue with, let's say, John Coltrane as a premier example. As a fan, I have listened to the five pieces featured on Coltrane's *Blue Train* album hundreds of times. There exists an organic engagement occurring between form and function, tenor and tone, music and audience. Aristotle taught, and Garcia reminds, that the interplay without audience input is impossible. Needed are not merely sheets and scores—quick fixes that easily replicate outdated recipes—but rhythm, timing, beat, off-beat, histories, experiences . . . nuances that inform and transform thinking. Anything less produces the same old superficial pieces that depend largely upon a type of rhetorical veneer resembling solutions.

Three decades ago, researcher Molefi Kete Asante produced breakthrough scholarship in a landmark book titled, *The Afrocentric Idea* (Temple University Press, 1988). As a young communication scholar, I was impacted greatly by Asante both as a rhetorician and person. His work inspired my publication titled, "African American rhetoric and the 'profession'" (*Western Journal of Communication,* Volume 57, Spring 1993). Asante argued that knowledge is placated when artifacts produced by non-Whites (speeches, songs etc.) are evaluated critically from a Eurocentric paradigm. Asante stated, "My work has increasingly constituted a radical critique of the Eurocentric ideology that masquerades as a universal view in the fields of intercultural communication, rhetoric, philosophy, education, anthropology, and history." At the time, his ground-breaking research challenged the dominant paradigm in social sciences research, in general, and in communication literature, in particular. The fact that critical ideologies don't work for all peoples placed a demand upon scholars to seek alternative perspectives. Borrowing from theories advanced by Asante, I advocated that rhetoric produced during church-sponsored mass meetings during America's civil rights years produced a robust localized rhetoric that included history, present, rhythm, and timing. The paucity of scholarship emphasizing such rhetoric produced "A curious footnote that raises some interesting questions" in communication scholarship. Asante et al., and now Garcia, are advancing similar questions: Why seek traditional approaches void of nuances that offer little potential to address health disparities?

Despite her exigencies, I still believe in America. However, if this is truly *the land of the free and the home of the brave,* more than people must be liberated. Thoughts, ideas, and the way meaning is constructed must endure a radical shift. Naysayers may say such a paradigm change is impossible and cannot be accomplished. Don't tell that to a group of 1960's Black doctors in Oakland, California. Only with such radicalism can this country qualify to be the proverbial *Beacon on a hill*—a global model for how doctors are trained and ought to treat folks.

Garcia is relentless in his pursuit of the truth that without a hunger for history, medical statistics will repeat disparities through the trite presentation of convention papers that do little more than appease the sensibilities of those committed to maintaining the status quo.

Foreword

As I complete this writing—February 28, 2019—I am mesmerized by an interview on the *Today Show*. Three innocent black men tell their harrowing story of a wrongful murder conviction that landed them in prison. When a Cleveland, Ohio salesman was murdered in 1975, an eyewitness testified that the three men were responsible. Upon conviction, Kwame Ajamu (then Ronnie Bridgeman), and brothers Wiley and Ricky Jackson, were sentenced to death based on the testimony of Edward Vernon. In 1980, due to a technicality, their sentences were commuted to life, but they would spend a collective total of over 100 years in prison before the eye witness admitted that he had lied to police authorities. When *Today Show* anchor, Craig Melvin, noted that the men did not seem angry or bitter, Ajamu responded that while he had forgiven Vernon for lying, he was in fact very angry and extremely bitter, not at an individual, rather at a system. Ajamu says he is angry over: *What is being perpetuated by a system by people we trust.*[1]

With one statement from a convicted killer now set free, the eerily similar parallels ought to serve as a warning for institutions that elevate traditional practices over dis-

---

1 The story of the men is the subject of a book, *Good Kids, Bad City* by Washington Post writer Kyle Swenson. New York: Picador, a trademark used by Macmillan Publishing Group (2019).

parities. As someone once stated, "If all you see is what you see, you don't see all there is that needs to be seen."

As Garcia rightly notes in this important work, jazz great Thelonious Monk found the true meaning of his music located "in the cracks" between the black and white piano keys. The unsophisticated, yet profoundly satisfying, symbolism constitutes a rhetoric that speaks to: simple, not easy; sensible, not sensational; alternative, not traditional; material, not delusional. That group of Oakland doctors demonstrated such in the care of their patients. Solutions to complicated issues are often incongruent, in the cracks, yet staring us in the face. They are not scripted or prescript. And to the horror of this rhetorician, they are not symmetrically poetic or logically binary. That's what makes this work so damn difficult. That's what makes this work of supreme value to the construction of meaning on health disparities.

Turn the album over Garcia. I wanna hear *Side B*.

Enrique D. Rigsby, Ph.D.

President, Rick Rigsby Communications

International Motivational Speaker, Minister & Best-Selling Author of *Lessons from a Third-Grade Dropout*

Part One

Framing Solutions

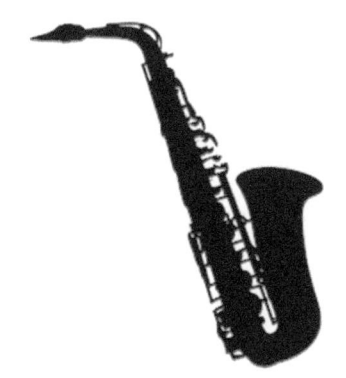

1
John Henry is Dead

There is an old folktale about John Henry, a mighty strong former slave, who beat a steam engine with his strength and determination, and then dropped dead. I try to imagine a reason someone might want to beat a steam engine. I recall an event where Jesse Owens raced a horse and wonder if John Henry's contest with the steam engine was along those commercial lines. To beat a steam engine seems an artificial, inhumane (unhuman!) exercise. The inhumanity smacks of allowing Black men with syphilis to go untreated during the antibiotic era of modern medicine in order to observe the natural progression of the disease. The "disease," I suppose, could be construed to mean either the syphilis, or the allowing of syphilis. That John Henry had to compete against a steam engine is disturbing, independent of our modern catastrophe of health disparities based on race.

Black boys, for example, are considered older than they are, and treated as such. So, a nine-year-old is treated like he's twelve; a twelve-year-old is shot dead within seconds; a teenager is tried as an adult.... As the father of a teenage Black boy, and as a sensible human being, I'm worried. This reminds me of the undergraduate classroom discussions with my Afro-American Literature professor, Barbara Christian, in the 1980s when she talked about chattel in the context of Afro-American novels from slavery to the present, culminating in a new novel, *The Color Purple*. This sort of inhumane treatment can be exacted upon chattel, and, it's clear from our reality, upon owned people. What's at hand here, then, is an attempt to convince someone who doesn't already agree that John Henry is human, and is precious, on those grounds alone.

I watched a recent documentary about Jackie Robinson. He died in 1972, when he was fifty-three years old. Coincidentally, I'm fifty-three years old. Robinson looked old to me in the months before he died. I don't suppose I look as old now as he did then. I could be wrong about this, as I don't see things the way others see them. I was eight years old, in the third grade, when Jackie Robinson died, though I was not conscious of either Jackie Robinson or John Henry. As a child, I'd always heard about Robinson as a figure in the remote past. He was the first Black player to play Major League Baseball in America. (Each time I hear this, I can't help but wonder who the first White player was.) My favorite line in August Wilson's play, *Fences*, comes when Troy responds to Rose and Bono about the caliber of baseball players in the segregated Negro Leagues: "Hell, I know some teams Jackie Robinson couldn't even make!"

Viola Davis said about August Wilson during an interview, "He was our griot." August Wilson died young. At sixty. Liver cancer. He smoked. That must have been it.

The best man at my wedding died young, too. He loved butter and ice cream, and had been obese since his adolescence. He sometimes noted with enthusiasm some of the early heights of his blood glucose levels. Near the end, as I struggled to convince him to eat less butter and more vegetables, he quipped, "I only eat things that had parents," a line I believe he took from a *Seinfeld* episode when Elaine teased Jerry about ordering a salad at a steak house. In a final, desperate attempt to save my best man's life, I noted that Luther Vandross, the reigning soul singer, had just died at the age of fifty-four, and that Minnesota Twin's baseball player, renowned slugger and centerfielder Kirby Puckett, who would leap above the outfield wall to snatch away a certain homerun, had recently died at the age of forty-five. As I tried to proceed, my best man, annoyed, interrupted my chronicle and said, "Oh, let's not list all the fat Black men who died."

I understand that it's important to tease apart rich fat deaths from the poor ones—thin or fat. And then it's important to tease further and further. When totaled, however, I'm left with the weight of excess deaths of Black people. Among many other publications, the 16th United States Surgeon General, David Satcher, MD, Ph.D., wrote a 2005 *Health Affairs* article, "What If We Were Equal? A Comparison of The Black-White Mortality Gap in 1960 And 2000," where he discussed the excess deaths for Black people that was 83,570 above what would have been expected if they had experienced mortality at the rate of White people.

If I consider that some of this excess is related to behaviors, like my best man's, that include an unhealthy diet, or else, cigarette smoking, other drug use, complications of obesity, trauma, cancer, and so forth, I understand that Whites suffer these same conditions. In fact, Black excess deaths notwithstanding, when considering the health of everyone, according to the World Health Organization, the United States ranked at #37, between Costa Rica and Slovenia, when compared with the other countries in the world. [That we pay far more than any other country in the world for this poor health is food for a different discussion. The combative discourse surrounding such calculations is not very interesting. The point—the U.S. pays way too much for what it gets—however, should not be lost.] Naturally, when—if!—we turn our attention to disparities based on race, such calculations are more oppressive.

I heard that one of my closest friends from childhood, Peewee, was stabbed to death during a misunderstanding over crack cocaine while I was an undergraduate student at Berkeley. Later, I heard that another friend was stabbed to death at a party where he encountered some rival teenagers. All of these teenagers had lived ordinary lives in Stockton. Like me. We rode our bikes, played basketball, watched Eddie Murphy movies at the mall, went to house parties on weekends. I returned home to Stockton recently and drove passed my old house where I saw another childhood friend. I stopped to chat with him. He said that he was proud of me for becoming a doctor, for "making it out." I smiled and dismissed any difference between us that he tried to highlight. We discussed a few who'd died: Johnny, Jeff, Who Boy. I'd heard that Dwight died. My friend said, "Yeah, a heart attack." With my medical education, attempting to be one with my history and my present, I casually replied, "I thought it was a stroke." My childhood friend effortlessly said, "He's dead, aint he?" setting aside my medical education, entirely, and snatching me back to our adolescent cultural verbal sparring. He won again.

The killing of Trayvon Martin paralyzed me. If I ever were to write about him, I'd have to start with Emmett Till. What's so paralyzing is that Emmett Till, fourteen years old, was killed with impunity in 1955; and Trayvon Martin, seventeen years old, was killed with impunity in 2012. Fifty-six years later: the same story. I get the impressionistic feeling of a Latin American short story written by, say, Juan Rulfo, that takes place as if time, itself, has not occurred. When Black people are shot to death at an early age, the analysis of excess deaths is less related to butter and ice cream, to smoking and drinking, and more related to immutable reality. However, there exists a struggle that must be. Slaves in early America, for example, who struggled against slavery, died before the end of slavery. Still, the struggle was necessary.

John Henryism places the locus of the pathology on the patient, himself. This necessarily relocates the focus—a stealth move!—*away* from the social environment that places him with his only option (or requirement) to work harder, endure more. It places him at the bottom of human hierarchy, at the whim of whoever established, and maintains, this social reality through which John Henry must struggle. Otherwise, of course, the status quo would have to indict itself. This is not a reasonable hope for Black people. To be able to place the locus of the analysis on the patient requires that the one placing this locus has the power to do so. This is what we have in our national discourse dating back to … well, all the way back.

John Henryism is not all social, to be sure. It is political, imperial, economic, history, law enforcement, etc. I often make the penultimate argument that it is a financial error to allow disparities to persist because sicker people cost more money, and since Black and Mexican people are sicker, ergo, paying attention to their health outcomes could save some money. However, I don't write in order to make money for Wall Street investors. Once that argument is clear, which isn't at all difficult, I try to make the ultimate argument—the one that Toni Morrison makes in her novel, *Beloved*, when she employs the sermon of Baby Suggs, holy, in the clearing: "This is flesh I'm talking about here." Or else, what I tried in my last book, *On Race and Medicine*, when Kramer asks Jerry Seinfeld to bring back some Cubans from Florida. Jerry asked a clarifying question: "We're talking about people, right?" These arguments have already been made. They've already failed. But in the context of health disparities where the cost of U.S. healthcare, and the disparities based on race, are on the nightly news, I might have a window to make this case in economic terms, in particular now. And in moral terms, in particular, now.

Invoking John Henryism is to explain the variance in health outcomes between races in social, economic, and "racial" terms. But this distracts from what to do about the variance. That verb, "to do," is the one that's avoided in America at a high cost. Indeed, the cost in cash, services, and flesh is not too high for the unaffected, or worse, the perpetuators, to address this verb. Race, itself, is distilled as the variable that has plagued America since before its beginning.

Another friend of mine, the president of a college in northern California, invited me to hear a guest lecture at her campus one evening where I would listen to an esteemed sociologist speak. The speaker, a Harvard professor, reminded the audience of the data showing that married men live longer than unmarried men; and that unmarried women live longer than married women, who put up with their husbands! This sort of thing, nebulously understood to be "stress," can account for tangible physiologic differences in health outcomes between men and women. This can be extended to the health outcomes delta between Black and White people, I suppose. But once we understand at least this part, then what? Shouldn't these data, and the subsequent would-be comprehension, propagate some mechanism to help? Otherwise, why bother? If these data do not engender a mechanism to improve things, then closing the gap in health outcomes never really was the goal. I'm not talking about what people say, rather, about what they do. And what they don't.

Though I'm not at all religious, I have this Bible passage memorized: 1 John 3:18. "Dear children, let us not love with words or speech but with actions and in truth."

What of the other, *main*, health disparities? These are unrelated, entirely, to John Henryism. The low rate of mammography among Black women is unrelated to them trying to navigate American history in the abstract. Black men with unchecked prostate cancer are unrelated to steam engines and whistling at White women. *How* Black people are treated—and not treated—in American medicine is relocated to the margins of a discussion about Black men stressed out in west Chicago, salt pork as a flavorful ingredient in a pot of mustard greens, and the like. That is, if Black people with known diabetes do not get their blood glucose monitored, and controlled, to the same standard as White people with known diabetes, no clever literary allegory can relocate this gap in care—care that's available, good, and accessed based on the "race" of the individual patient. Rather, the rhetorical location remains with the healthcare "system." Of course, the United States has no healthcare system, which makes a discussion about our system an unreality.

The variables that result in health outcomes disparities based on race impact John Henry, who struggles mightily en route to his own demise. They impact everyone else, too, less capable than John Henry, who also, naturally, succumb. Then, John Henry or not, the everyday variables are upon Black people—strong, weak, otherwise—such that the group, when compared with a group of Whites, are sicker. This understanding is not about an individual John Henryesque mythic or practical figure, but about people.

The question about John Henryism necessarily invites serious people to struggle through the intricacies of race in medicine. A potent, deadly intersection between race and medicine exists. A Venn diagram. Some areas don't intersect or overlap. Some do, but are not so decipherable. Black medical students are more likely to return to their communities to deliver care. While this has been true ever since medical schools started graduating Black doctors, disparities persist. While more and more Black doctors is a good idea, this is not *the* answer. And since there are incongruously few Black doctors given the need for healthcare for Black patients, they *must* see non-Black doctors based on the simple arithmetic dearth of Black doctors. Naturally, educating White and Asian and Indian medical students who might take care of Black patients about their Shakespearean slings and arrows of outrageous fortune is crucial if disparities is to be seriously confronted. Of course, this confrontation has not yet been the goal. No required congruence between the doctor's and the patient's race is reasonable. I saw a Thai ophthalmologist when I had trouble with my eye. His daughter went to kindergarten with my son. I suppose I could have looked for a Mexican ophthalmologist, but I was friends with the Thai …. *Voilà*, this discussion is off and running in the wrong direction.

My friend, an English professor, prepared a speech on John Henryism for an academic conference. Our initial exchange about John Henryism reminded me of the beginning of a chess match where things move quickly as we rid ourselves of the pesky pawns until we get a chance at the substance of the match. I wondered if she planned to take James Baldwin's approach and worry about the moral decay of the oppressor? Would she recommend a stealth approach where John Henry can parry the affronts, like a boxer, and save himself for the 15th round of the Heavy Weight Championship lest he tire himself out too soon, and get knocked out before the end of the bout? A "rope-a-dope" that enabled Muhammad Ali to knock out George Forman when I was a child? Or will she describe a Greek Tragedy that ends with the inevitable death of John Henry, despite our best efforts, the way Billie Holiday sounds sorrowful because she is sorrowful, and there's no getting around it? Our only hope, now, is to get through the sorrow.

2

Poor

I'd only met my father, a jazz trumpeter, three or four times before he died from an overdose of heroin. His sister remembered me, and has intermittently kept in touch through the decades since he died. She sends me notes: "Your cousin had a baby." I never knew any of these cousins. Indeed, I don't consider them cousins the way I consider my cousins. Still, I congratulate my aunt on the birth of a new cousin, and admire her interest in trying, against reason, to bind the "family" together. My aunt invited me to join her and one of these unknown cousins for drinks and appetizers at an Italian restaurant chain. Why not? I arrived and met my aunt and a much younger cousin from one generation below mine. Because I did not know these people who gave rise to me, I was unaware of any of the characters beyond my unknown father. I understood a profound sense of fatherlessness with these people. This cousin noted that several of *her* uncles and cousins were in prison for a wide variety of crimes. In order to keep the conversation going, I contributed that the men from my maternal lineage, starting with my grandfather and all of his brothers, my uncles, and my cousins, had all been to prison. Except me. The young second cousin who'd just met me a few minutes earlier interrupted and said, "Wow. You had it bad on both sides." I had considered that bad people get together and sometimes have children. Until that evening, however, I hadn't yet considered that I was one of these children.

My colleague from India, a pediatrician, and her husband, finishing up his Ph.D. in electrical engineering at Stanford, entertained me as I regaled them with colorful afternoons of Stockton, my poor city. Tales of a smart, aimless boy. I'd woven in a story about a friend from rural China who was discovered as a gifted child by the government, and ultimately led astray to graduate school in humanities in far off lands. Canada. Then the United States. I recounted my own tenth grade visit to a nearby university during a large lecture when I asked a question about the low, but real, rate of pesticide resistance among insects when spraying crops. This captured the attention of the agriculture dean who encouraged me to apply there in the coming years. This friendly exchange with my Indian friends had always been headed to my labyrinthine question about what would have happened to me if I had been a poor smart boy in, say, Calcutta. Still me; but there, and not in Stockton. Would the Indian government, like the Chinese government, have noticed a smart kid like me? The Indian pediatrician patiently allowed me to finish my everlasting, feline question. She was patient with me. Her restless engineer husband wasn't so patient. When I finally finished, she leaned forward a little and said, "I understand what you're asking, completely. But the real question is whether you will eat today."

Talk about race in medicine quickly, and necessarily, merges with talk about class. It then becomes *only* about poverty. "Improve healthcare for all" is an error in pragmatics because the difference between good healthcare and poor healthcare is a determined, enduring difference. It's also an error in arithmetic because if healthcare is improved equally for everyone, the difference will persist. Of course, this difference in health*care* is altogether different from good health *outcomes* and poor health *outcomes*. Someone clever will say that *we* might improve health outcomes for all *while* we improve health outcomes for the bottom even more. This breadth of mutual ascendency will result in general improvements for all, and will especially improve things for the bottom. Someone else, less clever, will respond to the call in error: "Rising tides lift all boats."

I'll smile.

I'll wonder about this "we," desperate to lift all boats. Desperate to lift the bottom. Where have "we" been? What took us so long to get here? What, now, brings us forward? Have we met? Do we know each other? When is our next get-together? What will we achieve then? When will this elevating work be done? Aren't all of these boats equally at the surface already? Or does this "we" mean to lift boats that have already sunk to the bottom? By what means? (Let me stop this line of self-inquisition here, mindful of a quote by James Carville during a presidential election of yore between Hillary Clinton and Barack Obama when Bill Richardson was referred to as a Judas because he did not support his friend, Hillary Clinton. The newscaster, quizzical, asked Carville, "Doesn't that make Hillary a Jesus figure?" James Carville dismissed the inquisitor in a sneering twang as only James Carville can sneer: "You never want to take these metaphors too far.")

I'll prod my friends' torment to morph every discussion about race into the more palatable discussion about class. That is, a poor White kid from an eastern Kentucky holler, in the end, can make it, we are taught as children. *Whether* he makes it isn't quite the plot in the American narrative.

I naturally enjoy discussions about class. I'm reminded of a late-night shift I had with an ER doctor, a Black man, when we bantered about our mutually exclusive, yet analogous, depressed childhoods. The ER doctor said about his childhood in South-Central Los Angeles: "We weren't poor. We were upper-lower-class!"

I have more homework to do on the class front, I admit. My deeply religious friend, who hasn't totally given up on me yet, tells me that Jesus addressed poverty, but did not solve for it. In fact, she notes that He didn't even try. I worry, then, that if Jesus didn't (or wouldn't) eradicate poverty, we will fall short. On the other hand, against logic, I'm open to the idea, or to the struggle, at least, even if I can't count on its corporeal reality.

The term "Structural Competence" is an emerging couple of words that replaces "socio-economic status," a couple from an earlier American discourse that evokes nostalgic college sociology lectures connoting the social location of someone's health risk: good or bad. Examples from this new language generally include an uninsured homeless man from, say, Oaxaca, with difficulty navigating the public transportation system of a big city. Or else he lives homelessly in a transportation desert that conjures images of food deserts in, say, Detroit, devoid of abundant grocery stores with fresh central California vegetables.

McDonald's is nearby.

The arc of such discussions of poverty at medical conferences, or in medical and social scientific publications, necessarily leads to a would-be mandate that medical students and residents training in family practice, internal medicine, and, to a lesser extent, pediatrics, not to mention psychiatry, should be overtly trained to take care of the poor Oaxacan far from home. And they should offer this care in his Mesoamerican Spanish. (This will be especially difficult if the Oaxacan speaks a primeval Zapotecan language. Let's hope he speaks his conqueror's Spanish.)

Humanity is implied for college students interested in medicine; for medical students, proper, en route to residency training; and for medical doctors, practicing already, throughout our careers. Whether we practice adjacent to Beverly Hills or on Chicago's west side makes no difference to medicine's requisite humanity. Indeed, humanity among doctors is not even implied, but is plain, evident to anyone either inside or outside of medicine. I'm not talking about money in medicine (yet). Rather, I'm talking about listening to a man's heart and hearing no sound.

The push for such social education to be included as a critical part of medical education is to argue that no such education—or not enough of it—takes place at the moment. Of course, such education is already upon us.

Integrated, at times; peripheral, at other times. The argument, then, is that more and better education about the social and structural contributors to disease, and to health, ought to be further included as integral to medical education, and not as afterthoughts, ghettoized in a throwaway lecture in a throwaway semester, in a voluntary noon conference with free pizza, or as incidental teaching points, dependent upon the teacher, entirely.

Step aside hepatocellular pathology! Make room for the poor.

"Structural Competence" is a slight of hand replacement for "Cultural Competence," which, itself, is a simple hoax that, even if possible, would only solve for cultural incompetence. What's needed to address overt disparities in health outcomes is *actual* competence.

"Structural" is a term diffuse to the point that no one, at all, comes to mind. I mentioned this construct to a cardiologist in a discussion about teaching medical school students about health outcomes disparities based on race. The cardiologist said, "Wait a minute. If you're telling me that poor people are sicker than rich people, I already know that. I don't need yet another medical journal article to tell me that one." Of course, telling any audience that poor people have predictably worse health outcomes, and that poverty, and its accoutrements, require attention before any hope can be realized, would only make sense if the audience didn't already know this. Then something else is necessary for the speaker. Being correct, as Aristotle notes about *logos* in *The Art of Rhetoric*, isn't enough to persuade the audience.

I was enthusiastic about attending a lecture about race for parents at an exclusive, elite high school. The esteemed speaker built his lecture with cinder blocks of everyday people of any color innocently being left out of ordinary society. "Car ignitions are made for right-handed people. Desks, too, are for righties. What are some other examples of how left-handed people are unwittingly biased against?" The speaker then talked about "unconscious" bias. Exasperated by then, I raised my right hand and said, "I'm more interested in *conscious* bias." The seasoned speaker countered in agreement and said that he preferred to use "implicit bias," to placate me.

Placating me isn't possible.

Shortly after the parent lecture, I noticed "implicit bias" appearing in medical discourse about health disparities. Such ideas reorient the audience to a particular doctor's actions, or inactions, to wholly explain differences in health outcomes between groups of people from different races. Sometimes when I tell someone about disparities in health outcomes between the races, he asks, "Why is that?" Certainly, there is nothing *implicit* about the centuries of worse outcomes based on race. These worse outcomes are not at all implied, but are actual.

The preacher momentarily turns his back to the pews and preaches to the choir during one of his crescendos because the choir needs to understand what he's saying when they sing. The pews, too, are important in gospel music.

I've spoken to some medical school deans about an academic design to graduate new doctors dedicated to decreasing disparities between races. But this cannot effectively be taught in medical school the way, say, histology is taught. The professors are exquisitely qualified in scientific fields. Histology tests are easy to grade. But education about race and disparities can't be easily graded as answers on a bubble-in scan sheet because they can't be proxies for concretized health outcomes for Mexicans with lower-leg amputations from diabetes or for Black people with sustained high blood pressure against which their hearts try hard to beat until they finally fail. These students, the deans note, must arrive at medical school already interested in this sensibility, the way they are interested in achieving good histology grades. To be sure, pre-medical students are sensitive to race and other social constructs as they submit their applications to medical schools. Nevertheless, persistent disparities in health outcomes between races exist. Blindness, amputations, heart failure, advanced breast cancer, hypertension unchecked. To look to eager, well-meaning medical students as *the* solution is an anemic distraction when the bulk of disparities rests in life outside of the ordinary clinical exchange.

The poor immigrant has different problems than Black people who have been in America for four hundred years, or Mexicans and Native Americans who have been here even longer, from before the beginning. The approach to helping these disparately sicker groups is different. The approach cannot be to tease apart each with words. A clash of possible terms serves to distract attention away from tangible progress, in any case. The homeless don't get homes; the hungry don't get food; the Black man with chest pain doesn't get a cardiologist. I remember a college meeting in the 1980s where Black students clashed for hours over the name of their would-be organization: Black Student Union v. Afro-American Student Union? I didn't attend the meeting because I didn't have standing, but heard from my roommate who exited early, when the meeting deteriorated into a discussion about behaviors in ancient Greece when discussing Black Greek-letter fraternities on campus. I don't recall the tangible results of the timeless meeting among my undergraduate classmates.

I'm afraid none emerged after all of the words—puffs of hot air—were exchanged.

If the audience already knows what's being said in a speech or a medical journal article, then what will make it *do* anything to help? The verb "to do" is the reduction sauce needed once the speeches and articles and data boil down. The intended audience, itself, has become a great interest of mine in the last few years. The best man at my wedding, a professor of classical rhetoric, noted that *the audience* is the most important part of any persuasive communication. I already know that being correct is not enough. Being a great speaker, too, is not enough. There is a requisite interplay with the audience. A jazz, as it were, where the listener's role is a more important element than the speaker or his speech. I've been exploring the intended audience from various angles. This is why I look to jazz, more than, say, classical music, when I consider a literary audience, a persuasive argumentative speech, the tangible outcomes of modern medicine, which remain worse for some races when compared with others. People who pay for healthcare—Medicare, Medicaid, private insurance companies, employers, everyday people—are missing from the conferences on health disparities I sometimes attend.

I'm generally crafty when avoiding questions about the intended audience when I discuss my own writing. I start my yarn with a quote by playwright August Wilson's dramatic claim that he wrote for an "audience of one." Himself. That he then took his plays to the stage is not altogether a *non sequitur*. I like Emily Dickinson, too, who actually did put her poems in a closet. I also note Nobel Prize-winning poet Joseph Brodsky's proclamation that he wrote to an audience comprised of writers from antiquity: Ovid, Virgil, Horace, Suetonius, among the others. My best man, the rhetorician, noted about Brodsky's intended audience of antiquity: "Those people have already read all they're going to read by Brodsky." I typically end my parry about the intended audience with my own readings of Dostoyevsky's *Notes from Underground*, which led me to *Crime and Punishment*, and then *The Brothers Karamozov* when I finished medical school and point out that Dostoyevsky could not have had a poor Mexican from future Stockton in mind when he wrote his Russian literature in the mid-1800s.

This sly deflection doesn't work well in medicine where tangible disease and avoidable excess death is at the heart of the discourse.

Who is the intended audience when writing about would-be solutions to centuries of health outcomes disparities between American races? We try to keep each other motivated, vigilant, those of us without the power to enact solutions. But it's as if we're talking to the air.

Alas, these payers of healthcare, these everyday people, should not only be the intended audience, but part of the collective of speakers. They would bring *ethos*.

My friend, an allergist, told me about his mobile asthma clinic that successfully treats poor children around the city. This mobile asthma clinic is both clinically and financially successful. I enjoyed his narrative until the end when he mentioned that the city officials plan to terminate the project. I asked why the officials would terminate a clinically and financially successful project that helps poor children breathe and keeps them from going to the ER where the cost is high, and when the reason they are in the ER is because their routine asthma treatment has failed. My friend clarified that the city officials were not aware of the program's success. I said, "I have an idea: Why don't you tell them?"

3

Marble Rye

My tenth grade Physical Anthropology textbook displayed a diagram of the evolution of man. I recall some prehistoric version of a monkey, then Lucy, perhaps, evolving in sketches to more advanced primates, Peking, Neanderthal, Cro-Magnon, and so forth, with the final sketches culminating in an upright White male: the height of human evolution, based on the scientific evidence, we were all taught.

The Last Samurai is a movie about ancient Japanese sword warriors starring Tom Cruise. Set in the late 1800s, maybe the movie was not about Japanese sword warriors, but about the requisite American intervention around the world in the guise of Tom Cruise. I saw the movie a long time ago, so I don't remember the details now, and can't recall whether the last Samurai was the Japanese character, or, in some middle adolescent literary effort, was meant to be Tom Cruise. What struck me then, and now, as I think about Tom Cruise as the movie's lead, conflating the title with his name, is that if we, the intended audience, are to understand Japanese antiquity, and its decay, we had better do this *only* insofar as the arc of Japanese history can be understood on behalf of White people. Tom Cruise, then.

This is not quite the "White gaze" Toni Morrison explained in an interview as she noted that her characters are not to be seen insofar as they represent props in support of White life, only significant because they create a reality with a White audience in mind. Her characters are to be understood independent of White people. Morrison noted that Ralph Ellison did not have a Black intended audience in mind—her, for example—when he wrote *Invisible Man*. Ellison explained things to a White audience that would not need to be explained to a Black audience. That is, Ellison's narrator was not invisible to Toni Morrison. She saw him clearly.

But with *The Last Samurai*, we don't see the Japanese characters through the eyes of Tom Cruise. Rather, we see them *because* they support a story about White people.

Tom Cruise.

Japanese history can be understood in the absence of Whites; but its worthiness can only be measured against Cruise's yardstick.

I saw *Dances with Wolves* when I was nearing the end of medical school. It's a movie about Lakota Native Americans starring Kevin Costner. Well, not *about* Lakota, but about Costner. What struck me most about that movie, aside from the foretelling of the impending genocide, was that I could not recall ever seeing long black hair at the fore of such a big movie. I paid more attention to the Lakota than to Costner, which was difficult, given the American narrative. In fact, I had been considering growing my own black hair long. I'd noticed U2 lead singer, Bono's, hair by then. I wasn't certain that this would work out well as a medical student. Nevertheless, I let my hair grow. I had not yet realized how difficult it would be to grow the front hair so that it would be, in the end, longer than the back hair, though would appear even, like the Lakota or like Bono. Because I'm Mexican, once I let my hair grow long, below my shoulders, during my pediatric internship the year after medical school, I looked like a Native American. Maybe Lakota? Maybe Comanche? Maybe Mexican?

I enjoyed *McFarland*, a movie about Mexican farm workers' children who ran on their high school cross country team in central California. I was delighted to see that these Mexicans, who reminded me of myself as they academically meandered through high school, became California State cross country champions in this movie starring requisite Kevin Costner.

I like Kevin Costner movies.

By the time I saw *Windtalkers,* a movie about the Navajo, starring Nicholas Cage, I realized that I had not really thought about Tom Cruise or Kevin Costner when I saw their respective movies. But with *Windtalkers,* I started thinking about why a movie apparently about the use of the Navajo language during World War II to help defeat Japan, unable to break the "code" of the Navajo language, would *require* Nicholas Cage. Of course, this construct is about money. A bankable actor. Cage then, though evidently not now.

I watched a documentary that discussed race in movies. A White man with the power to green light a movie was asked what the budget would be for a movie with the same script starring Black actors when compared with White actors. I don't recall the exact quote, but he said something like, "If it were a movie with, say, Denzel Washington and Halle Berry (who had won the Academy Award for Best Actress by then, I think) and, say, Robert De Niro and Meryl Streep, the budget would be… *(pause)*… half." The Green Light man didn't appear sinister. Didn't appear at all oppressive in his casual cloths at his beach home. Maybe he wore shorts and a T-shirt. He sounded utterly qualified, and spoke with envious indifference. Maybe it wasn't De Niro and Streep. Either way, I understood his point.

But this movie reality is not only about money.

I'm not talking about white actors playing black or brown characters. I recall an Asian American Studies course where we learned that Katherine Hepburn, with Scotch Tape above her eyes, played a Chinese peasant who stood up to Japanese invaders in *Dragon Seed*. John Wayne played Genghis Khan, builder of the Mongol Empire several centuries before John Wayne won the American West. Mickey Rooney played a cartoon, Mr. Yunioshi, in *Breakfast at Tiffany's*. David Caradine played Kwai Chang Caine in the TV series, *Kung Fu*. I don't suppose it was all that bad to have a Filipino actor play a Mexican in *Stand and Deliver*. (Were there no Mexicans available?) Maybe a Filipino, Leah Solanga, playing a young Vietnamese woman in the musical, *Miss Saigon*, was also not too much of a stretch. I read that the wonderful Welsh actor, Jonathan Pryce, who played the Vietnamese character, The Engineer, was more offensive. I wonder: Offensive to what end?

I prefer Bruce Lee in *The Chinese Connection* when he read the "No Dogs and Chinese Allowed" sign, flew into the air, kicked the sign off the wall, and, while levitating still higher, kicked the sign again, splintering it into shards of indecipherable wood to Kevin Costner in *Hidden Figures* tearing down the Colored Only signs that disallowed Taraji P. Henson the ability to urinate freely. Lee was nationalistic, which I prefer as an audience.

Cry Freedom is a movie by Richard Attenborough about South African anti-apartheid activist Stephen Biko, played by young Denzel Washington, as understood through Kevin Kline. *The Last of the Mohicans* stars my favorite, Daniel Day-Lewis. *The Last King of Scotland* is about Idi Amin, the Ugandan dictator, who is understood because of the White character. I can't remember what he did in the movie beyond being White. *The Soloist,* starring Jamie Foxx, is understood through Robert Downey, Jr. *42* is a movie about Jackie Robinson, starring Harrison Ford. *The Man Who Knew Infinity* is a movie about a remote Indian mathematician, played by the mighty Dev Patel, who is interesting only insofar as he interacts with Jeremy Irons in England. *Silence* is a movie set in Nagasaki during the 1600s, starring *Spiderman's* Andrew Garfield and Adam Driver, Han Solo's son. Matt Damon starred in *The Great Wall*. In response to accusations of White saviors required by Chinese people, Damon pleaded that it was a monster movie, and not a movie about White people saving Chinese people. "It's about monsters." He urged the audience to see the movie before charging him, yet again, as a Bourne Supremacist. I don't believe anyone in the accusing audience took his advice. Or else, *Invictus*, a movie concerned with race in the post-Apartheid era of Nelson Mandela in South Africa, starring Matt Damon alongside perennial Morgan Freeman.

American Gangster featured Russell Crowe in parallel with Denzel Washington. I enjoyed another movie starring Washington, along with Gene Hackman, *Crimson Tide*. My favorite part is when Washington did not recognize Captain Hackman's authority. I wondered about how Hackman, unfettered, was able to slap Washington. Sydney Poitier declined to allow a White man to slap him without Poitier returning a definitive slap in the Rod Steiger movie, *In the Heat of the Night*. Though I didn't see it, I like the title of the follow up movie better, *They Call Me Mr. Tibbs*.

I enjoyed *Glory*, a movie about a Black regiment in the U.S. Civil War, with Denzel playing a subordinate character to the star of the movie, Matthew Broderick, whom I enjoyed on Broadway in *The Producers*, a play about Jewish producers. I don't know if Broderick is Jewish; I know he's not Black.

I suspect that these Washington movies required White actors in order to be bankable to Green Light men. I notice that other Crowe and Hackman movies don't require a Black actor.

I did not see Brad Pitt as Achilles in *Troy*. My colleague, a pediatric endocrinologist, from Greece had no words for this one. Eye-rolling and a grimace clarified things for me. I suppose Greeks could be White. I suppose Pitt could pass as Greek. I think she was offended that Pitt played Achilles.

I didn't see *The Godfather Part II* in the theater. I was too young back then. Although, I cannot separate times in my memory that do not contain this movie now that I've seen it too many times to count. That is, I've enjoyed many movies about White people throughout my life. Most movies, in fact. I recalled reading the novel, *One Flew Over the Cuckoo's Nest,* near the end of high school. I don't know if I saw the movie then. I did buy it much later, when I was traveling often, and wanted to watch movies. I purchased the DVD. (I am not yet confident in my ability to stream.) My favorite line is when McMurphy says to the voluntary mental hospital patients, "Come on you nuts." I was too young to understand *The Deer Hunter* when I saw it, but understood that I was watching some serious acting. I loved *Tootsie*. I didn't think that Cher was not Italian in *Moonstruck*. Of course, that second, harder slap across Cage's face is the defiance I love about Cher. I consider Meryl Streep in *Sophie's Choice* as the gold standard for acting. When I wonder if, say, Viola Davis or Denzel Washington, or Meryl Streep, for that matter, has done a good job, I compare the acting to Streep in *Sophie's Choice*. I missed many movies when I was in college and medical school. I heard about Daniel Day-Lew in *My Left Foot* many years after he'd won an Academy Award for Best Actor. I've seen Irish plays on Broadway and in Los Angeles, to be sure, were not meant for an audience comprised of a poor Mexican from Stockton. Our mutual humanity, however, was plain, immediate. I appreciated Russell Crowe's determination in *Gladiator*. I could not have been prepared for *Winter's Bones*, a movie about Ozark Whites and adolescent determination. Before I knew who she was, I recognized Jennifer Lawrence's portrayal of a hero as my own. I watch *A Few Good Men* every few weeks, as it airs regularly, it seems, on weekends. *Billy Elliot* is my favorite because he had no reason to hope, which, in any case, didn't deter him. I was nervous as a child when I saw *Jaws*. I believe I became teary as a child during *Kramer vs. Kramer*. Many years later, as an adult, I was afraid to watch *The Silence of the Lambs*. I did not see it at the theater. I watched it later, at home, with the lights on. I trained at the hospital in

Chicago where Harrison Ford in *The Fugitive* worked. I found the cerebral *Quiz Show* a pleasure. *Fargo*! I identified with the poor, smart young man in *Good Will Hunting*. I was bedazzled by Marcia Gay Harden in *Mystic River*. Like so many others, I stopped drinking merlot after I watched *Sideways*. I struggled with the ending of *The Accidental Tourist*. I liked the math in *Moneyball*. And Jonah Hill! I use lines from *My Cousin Vinny* in my everyday speech. During the time when I traveled often, I took the opportunity to watch movies I'd missed, and sensed that I should have them at the ready when talking. I watched some of the old Pacino movies until I found *Dog Day Afternoon*. This seemed more than a movie to me. In an embarrassingly haphazard, if not cursory, forage through movies (and novels) that I'd missed while getting educated in college and medical school, I stumbled into *Network*. Had it not been for my commensurate uncovering of Faulkner's *Absalom, Absalom!*, Gabriel García Márquez's *One Hundred Years of Solitude*, and Jorge Luis Borges's *Ficciones*, I would not have been prepared for the narrative in *Network*. I appreciated the artistic importance of *Casablanca*, *On the Waterfront*, and *Citizen Kane*. I didn't once consider that Gene Hackman required a Mexican actor in order for *Unforgiven* to mean something to me. I did not consider that the great Paul Giamotti required Jamie Foxx or Will Smith as a vehicle for his humanity. I didn't see the need for a miscellaneous Black actor in *Network* or *Good Will Hunting* in order for me to recognize the particular humanity in White stories like, say, Dostoyevsky's Raskolnikov, or Edward Albee's *Three Tall Women*, was meant for me. I love *The Beauty Queen of Leenane*. I don't need a Mexican *Billy Elliott* to be human.

I like these movies. These plays.

I identify with them.

I am not White.

This recognition of mine is not meant to be an exhaustive list of movies that reports past offenses of White actors in black face. It's not about Olivier as Othello. More qualified people have already done such forensic pieces. Rather, I'm interested in the habit of presenting narratives in forms that, to be sure, connote an expected—and understandable—inferiority for those of us who are not land-owning White males, the primogenitures in America. A habit that requires us to ask for approval to exist as full-bodied human beings.

I began thinking about race in these terms when I saw the *Seinfeld* episode with the marble rye. I was impressed that Jerry Seinfeld and Larry David didn't find it at all consequential to explain the significance of a marble rye to a Mexican who never would consider the bread. As a fan of *Seinfeld*, I accepted this to be a routine understanding of

Jewish people. Maybe I was wrong. Either way, I enjoyed the episode, entirely. I never did look into the significance of marble rye. (I imagine a television show that includes a tortilla without exposition about the intricacies and nuances that I naturally understand.) That is, Seinfeld and David were indifferent to whether an audience unfamiliar with marble rye could appreciate the comedy. An impressive nationalism in keeping with Bruce Lee's kick, and the shards from the exploding wooden sign.

Rick Rigsby, Ph.D. wrote a chapter about doctors' communication with patients in my last book. He chronicled a house call that his own pediatrician made when Rigsby and his brother were children. Another friend read this chapter and noted that while it was in a book about race and medicine, the chapter, itself, did not talk about race, *per se*. We called Rigsby to question this rhetorical move. Rigsby, always gracious, said about his chapter: "I'll have to go back and check, but I thought I mentioned Billy Dee Williams. White people don't sit around and talk about Billy Dee Williams. Those are Black people."

I am a doctor. I consider how our humanity, itself, can withstand the necessary invisibility in the face of human decay that health disparities bespeak.

My mother, a Mexican woman from central California, when returning from a drive across the border between California and Mexico in the 1980s, was paused by the Border Patrol at the point of reentry in San Diego. Among other things, the officer asked her who the president of the United States was. Nervous in the Californio-Mexican heat, she blurted out, "John Wayne." The Border Patrol officer laughed at her conflation of John Wayne and Ronald Reagan, and waived my mother back into California.

The best man at my wedding, a rhetorician with a Ph.D. from Berkeley, suggested that I go see the movie, *Crouching Tiger, Hidden Dragon*. "They have people flying through the air." I've always enjoyed Chinese martial arts movies since my early adolescence in Stockton, and had heard much about the critical reception the new movie received. I went to see *Crouching Tiger, Hidden Dragon*. Afterward, I called my best man and said, "I didn't know you meant they were *really* flying!" He said, "Yes. What did you think I meant?" He noted that the ending was not at all American. I noticed that, too, but didn't know what to make if it. I had not yet considered un-American movie endings.

I recall a movie from the 1980s, *A Soldier's Story*, about a Black Army regiment where the White characters were supportive. This began as Charles Fuller's Pulitzer Prize-winning play on Broadway, *A Soldier's Play*.

August Wilson's plays are located in Black characters. I like *Joe Turner's Come and Gone,* among the others. *Gem of the Ocean.*

I don't remember any White characters in Kasi Lemmons's movie, *Eve's Bayou.*

An old Black doctor told me that he would drive through the south with his classmates during the 1940s when he was in college and medical school. The carful of young Black scholars stopped at one place, then another, to find that they could only purchase food through the back door of a restaurant, and would have to drive away to eat it. Insulted, they'd drive to the next stop, then the next, defiant at each stop, declining to submit to the indignity. By nightfall, at the next stop, one of the students went up to the restaurant and was told what he had heard all day. He returned to the carful of young Black scholars and the old doctor to be said, "I'll have two chili dogs and an order of fries."

I have not seen *Green Book*, a movie about a White man who drives a Black man through the the American South. I heard this movie won an Oscar for Best Picture. I think I already know its essence. There is no White driver in the Best Actor category while the Black man rests in the Best Supporting Actor category in my version of reality. I hear that both actors are wonderful. I might not be able to stomach the movie, I worry. Maybe this is my loss. The price I pay for my defiance.

Decreasing health disparities can be argued on financial grounds such that investors can make some money. There are only two ways, more or less, to decrease the gap in health outcomes between the races: treat Black and brown people better, or treat White people worse. The latter is not a winning argument. Neither is the former, it appears. If the very reason any story, at all, is interesting is because it's *about* White people, and because it furthers their esteem, then I understand that discussions about decreasing health disparities must be argued on financial grounds such that Wall Street can make some money, and not on human decency grounds, which is a higher form of Aristotelian persuasion.

4

Distractions

―――•◦•●•◦•―――

Savion Glover stood on the stage between tap dances and silently stared at the audience. Sitting still, all of us, we stared back at him. I've seen him many times in the past, and am no longer surprised by his artistic choices as much as I am enchanted, captivated by what he does in the present, with each tap slide pause, not at all anticipating, let alone ready for, what might be next. Glover's present—in speech, tapping on stage, or walking toward Eighth Avenue, say, in the time between Saturday's matinee and night shows—whether tapping or pausing, is hearty. No one moved. Not Glover; not the other dancers; no one in the audience. There is a vent in the ceiling ticking, metered perfectly, with one of the blades hitting the metal cover of the air conditioner in the auditorium. This goes on for a long time, eternal in its representation, as Glover stands still staring at us. Is he thinking of the first step in his next opening? Is he resting after the thunderous piece he just finished? I looked around to see if someone was going to attend to the perfectly measured ticking, somehow, by turning off the air conditioner, perhaps, on the hot afternoon. Unlikely. I figured once Glover got started, the music, the thunderous tap dancing, the joyful atmosphere, itself, his arms flailing incongruent with his dreadlocks, would distract me from the tick ticking that, by now, cheapens the experience. My wife and I have seen Savion Glover many times—on Broadway in *Bring in 'Da Noise, Bring in 'Da Funk*, on Wilshire tapping in his socks!, in Chicago with the symphony, and everywhere else we could manage. We took our three children, this time, and sat in the front row at the university theater so that our children, whether they could, yet, appreciate Savion Glover, would know that we thought they ought to see him up close. I gently looked around, then up, to see if I could make sense of the repeating metered noise in the otherwise silent university theater. Nothing. I looked at Savion Glover standing on the stage and noticed his right foot imperceptibly moving, causing what I had initially thought was a misshapen fan blade hitting, perfectly, against something during the quiet of Glover's agenda. It was him! Perfectly. Then he danced again, moving more than just his right foot, imperceptibly. Arms and feet and dreadlocks flying in an eternal starburst.

Flipping through the channels, I stopped at a documentary about a public high school in northern California. I'd missed the beginning, but gathered that this was a predominantly Mexican high school with a poor academic record. The camera aimlessly panned the outdoor lunch tables filled with Mexican teenagers dressed as high school students. The narrator noted that the high school had a fifty percent dropout rate. I understood the indifferent camera pan and the narrator's statistical prediction about the foretold dropouts to mean that any random half of the students—not one particular Mexican—is what mattered in these data, in this panoramic view, and would drop out. I instantly recalled that we had 500 ninth graders at my high school a few cities over from the documentary city, where I graduated among 250 seniors. No one could have picked me out of a cafeteria pan during lunch as one of the future graduates. My own children live starkly different childhoods than mine. One hundred percent of the students graduate from their elite high school; and one hundred percent attend esteemed colleges and universities. My wife, our children, and I walked onto a different college preparatory high school where we considered sending our younger child. This was a Sunday, when the school was closed. The man who guarded the gate was not there the moment we drove up, so I parked the minivan and we walked through the campus to at least see the buildings. An educated man, I understood that our impromptu stopping by would need to be formally followed up. I tried to imagine the illustrious student body with our son sitting among them. Deep into the campus, a White woman with a limp saw us walking. She turned and faced our direction. We did not run. She finally reached us and asked how we'd gotten onto the campus. I told her. She said that it was a closed campus, and that we should have made an appointment for a visit. She motioned for us to follow her back to the front gate. She picked up the pace and motioned for us to hurry and follow her as she escorted us off of the private, illustrious campus. Naturally, I knew we didn't belong on campus. I even felt a little thrill that reminded me of the times I jumped over the barbed wire fence at my high school football games to avoid paying the entrance fee. I felt like I did during a basketball game as an undergraduate student at Berkeley when we were scheduled to play against UCLA during Reggie Miller's senior year. I'd heard that we had not beaten UCLA in twenty-five games. Or was it twenty- five years? I snuck into the gym too early, and was spotted by security because I was the only student in the seats while the television crew set up. He threw me out. Defeated, I headed back to my dorm to watch the game on TV. I passed a door with a large crowd of students who were to work as vendors inside the gym during the game.

At the precise moment I passed the crowd, the doors to the gym opened and the students rushed in, each stated their role as vendors: Hot dogs, soda, cotton candy.... Quickly, I jumped into the middle of the rushing crowd. When I reached the front, I looked at the guard and said, "Peanuts." I believe we won the game against UCLA, but I would need to verify this memory. I'm not suggesting that the hobbled woman treated us like criminals. Perhaps we were trespassing. Criminals, then. But for all their cries for diversity, I haven't gotten the sense that college prep schools find that we—a Mexican husband, a Black wife, three children of varying shades—do things differently. Sometimes we just show up unannounced, independent of their etiquette. Maybe this is wrong. They're in positions to judge when they see us. In our unplanned, unrehearsed, unapologetic visit, *we saw them*, too. We didn't send our son there. We didn't even apply. I don't suspect they wanted him.

I sat alone at a Thai restaurant in Scottsdale on a forgotten Monday night. I'd walked around the tony town looking for dinner after a day of business meetings. The sign in front: Jazz Every Monday from 6-9. I could hear the trio when I entered the front door and approached the hostess. She asked if I wanted a table in the main restaurant, or in the area where the jazz trio played. I chose the trio. She found a small table in the back of the close quarters with a few tables between me and the trio. I was minimally disturbed by a woman and her elderly parents sitting next to me. I thought they should eat quietly and listen to the jazz. A singer, who had been on a break when I arrived, rose from the crowd and sang a Sarah Vaughan song. The adults talked more, but I was able to disregard them once the Tom Kha Gai, along with the Sarah Vaughan, arrived. A party of six walked up to the hostess. She sat them at a large table, near the trio, in an empty part of the restaurant I had not noticed. Not the main dining room, and not the part where I sat, but deeper in, off to the side. The family walked around to the booth where the hostess sat them. They had a baby. The baby cried. I had not yet considered live jazz with a crying baby before then. I ate my soup and left the restaurant only partially satisfied.

I latched onto a family of Black physicians when I was in college. The patriarch was one of only two Black physicians to have served as the president of the California Medical Association. He was also the president of the National Medical Association, an organization of Black physicians established in 1895, when they could not join the American Medical Association, a White organization. Two of his children and several nieces and nephews were physicians. The family honestly absorbed me such that I would borrow the Volvo, stay at the house when they were away on vacation, and, finally, join them at births, graduations, weddings, family reunions, and deaths. My favorite was Uncle Jonathan, a professor at a local college. I sat next to him at every chance. I found his comedy both subtle and incisive. These were my favorite parts. Certainly, he was also serious and substantive. The elders grew up in segregated Charleston, South Carolina. They had recently driven through Charleston on a family trip home. While driving through The Citadel, Uncle Jonathan asked to stop the car. "Just stop." They pulled over and Uncle Jonathan got out, sat down on the grass, then rolled around. Laughing, the brothers recalled the time when Black people could not stand on the grass at The Citadel. Uncle Jonathan told me about a new, young Black professor who joined him on the faculty at the local college. As they prepared to walk across campus to lunch, or to a meeting, Uncle Jonathan said to the young Black professor, "Let me show you how to walk across campus." The young Black professor didn't understand. Uncle Jonathan explained, "Leave early because you have to stop and talk to every Black child you see from the time you leave to the time you arrive across campus. If you don't, they won't have any Black professors they can talk to. Plus, I had to leave early so I could talk to you."

I considered race, *per se*, in 1976, at the end of the sixth-grade, when we found that White students would be bused to our middle school the next year. This integration was the result of the Supreme Court decision, *Brown v. Board of Education of Topeka Kansas* in 1954, ten years before I was born. We left home early and walked the two miles to our middle school such that we arrived at the same time the buses unloaded the White children. Before this, we were Filipino, Black, Japanese, Mexican, and Chinese, for the most part, in south Stockton. This was around the time a White applicant, among others, was denied admission to medical school at the University of California at Davis. I went to college, and then to medical school, in the decade after the White student's Supreme Court challenge, *U.C. Board of Regents v. Bakke, 1978*. (By utter coincidence, I worked briefly with a Black doctor who said, "I'm the one who took Bakke's spot." We laughed, and quarreled about whether it was *his* spot. It turned out that it was his spot, according to the United States Supreme Court.) I would later meet the Chair of the UC Davis School of Medicine Task Force on Opportunities for Disadvantaged Students. We talked about health disparities based on race. The Task Force Chair recalled that many years earlier, while the case was being argued at the Supreme Court, he walked across campus with the big dean of the medical school. The big dean said that he was worried because all of the Black students were sitting together during lunch. The Task Force Chair looked around at the rest of the open area and asked the dean if he was worried that all of the White students were sitting together.

A White student at the University of California at Berkeley asked our sociology professor, Harry Edwards, "Where's the White counterpart to Michael Jordan?" Harry instantly redirected (and educated) the illustrious student: "Hell, where's the Black counterpart to Michael Jordan?" I don't want Miles Davis to be equal to White trumpet players. Or to Black ones, for that matter. Miles's notes are not equal. Neither do I want my brown son to be equal to White sons. No one ever fired overt racial slurs at me. No orchard overseer ever treated me as a set of arms good for picking cherries or apricots or anything at all. I had no sense that I was a minority the way the word applies to me now. I am a Mexican from central California who has never picked fruit outside of the produce section of a grocery store chain, living a reality oblivious to hierarchical power. The closest was during a dorm debate as an undergraduate at Berkeley when a White student said about my complaining about Ronald Reagan, or some such thing, "If you don't like it here, why don't you go back to where you came from?"

His grammar notwithstanding, I said, "Stockton? How would going back there help?" Yet, somehow, I cannot help but walk toward race. "I'm a race guy" is what August Wilson, the great playwright who chronicled ten decades of particular versions of reality for Black people that begins in the centuries before the twentieth, and will span for centuries after, offered during an interview on *60 Minutes*, when Ed Bradley, I think it was, asked Wilson if he was angry. Wilson told of an unarmed Black man on his front porch who was shot fifty-six times by the police, and of a White man who stood outside of the White House with a rifle threatening to shoot the president when the police talked him down. "Yes, I'm angry. A hundred yards from the leader of the free world and they talked him down; and they shoot an unarmed Black man fifty-six times." (Whether it's a free world, and whether he was its leader, is for another time.) In a different interview with Bill Moyers, Wilson said, "You can never transcend who you are."

My friend, a Pakastani physician, said, "When I came to America, I presented my patient on the first day of hospital rounds. The attending cut me off. 'You must state the age, race, and gender of each patient. This guides your thinking.' I thought about this and realized that I'd sound like an idiot back home if I said, 'This is a thirty-year-old

Pakistani male.' Everyone is Pakistani. We're in Pakistan! But, if that's how they do things in America, then OK." Another friend, a doctor who graduated from Stanford, and his wife, who also graduated from Stanford, then from law school at Harvard, both Mexican, bought an old house in a university neighborhood. They liked the idea of fixing it up so that they'd have a nice place to live; and so that they might resell it for a profit someday. During the escrow closing ceremonies, they noticed that the deed still stated "White Only." The escrow officer, apparently embarrassed, offered to remove that phrase. My friends declined. They wanted to keep it for their American records. They work with poor Mexicans in their respective fields and remind us of our humanity. Our possibility. Our decency. Our dignity. They embrace their deed the way a jazz artist embraces tragedy during a fantastic solo.

I visited my neighborhood grocery store, owned by a Nisei man, the year Vanessa Williams won the Miss America pageant. An old Black man waiting at the butcher counter engaged in repartee with the Black butcher, a twenty-two-year-old man who had worked in the Japanese family grocery store since he was twelve years old—initially as a stock boy, then the cash register, then the butcher counter. (Incidentally, he had a beautiful falsetto and sang lead in the defunct Baby Brother Band, a local group that would never make it big.) The old Black man noted that he watched the beauty pageant the night before on his old black and white television. He'd tuned in late, and only caught the part where the five finalists stood on stage before the audience. The old Black man noted that because his television was old, it needed time to warm up before he could see the picture clearly. During the warm up, the pageant host announced that for the first time in history there were two Black finalists among the five. The picture emerged and the old Black man could see the five finalists, but could not tell which two of the five were Black. The bottom three were eliminated, with the two Black contestants remaining, one who was to become Miss America, and the other the runner up. Still, the old Black man could not tell that there were any Black people, at all, on his black and white television. Vanessa Williams won the crown; and Suzette Charles was the runner up. The old Black man took the emcee at his word.

I planned a trip to New York to see some plays and listen to jazz at the Village Vanguard. Looking forward to catching up with some friends, I let them know I'd be there in the coming weeks. One friend, a Wall Street investment banker, looked forward to meeting, to seeing a musical, and to catching up. Another, an ACLU lawyer, said that she'd be away that week working on an education case in South Dakota. I think it had something to do with discrimination against Native Americans, but I'm not certain. I went to New York and enjoyed my stay. I saw whatever was on sale at the 50% Off TKTS counter. A musical, I'm sure. A drama or two. I think I saw *Cabaret* that time, starring Alan Cumming, who had won a Tony, among other awards, for his roll as the Master of Ceremonies in a previous production a decade earlier. When I returned to California, I called my ACLU friend and asked how her case went in South Dakota. Innocently, she replied that she didn't get much accomplished on the current case because neither White nor Lakota had yet been able to get over the Battle of Little Big Horn in 1876. I laughed, and took for granted that she was joking. She wasn't. She left South Dakota and returned to New York City without addressing the current case. I suggested that the next time she might plan to stay longer, and start the discussion before the Battle of Little Big Horn.

As an early adolescent, I heard one of the guys in the neighborhood say that Mama Cass choked to death on a ham sandwich. I did not question the accuracy of the report. I don't know how this point even made it into a discussion in my childhood neighborhood. We were Mexican, Filipino, Black, Chinese, and Japanese children such that The Mamas and the Papas were not part of our adolescent songbook in the mid-1970s. I think it must have been as part of a verbal tournament of insults about respective maternal obesity between two of the Black kids. I don't recall the details. Decades later, Mama Cass's daughter pointed out the pain she felt when this story circulated about her mother. This was, in fact, a hurtful fiction of the daughter's life. It was around this time that I'd begun to read interviews and nonfiction articles about Gabriel García Márquez. In one response about his magical realism he said that if he tells someone that he'd seen a flying elephant, he would not be believed. But if he told them that he'd seen seventeen flying elephants, this would be more believable than seeing just the one. Something like that. Maybe they were pink elephants. I didn't believe it; I didn't disbelieve it. I never thought about it again until I heard Mama Cass's daughter, who is around my age, note the cruelty of this popular version of her mother's death. I agreed, but didn't think much more about this. Many years later, while haphazardly searching for music from the Vietnam War era, which is burned in my head, as far as I can tell, as the soundtrack to *Forrest Gump*, I found "White Rabbit," by Jefferson Airplane, which I didn't understand. I added "For What It's Worth," by Buffalo Springfield. My daughter, in high school at the time, had discovered *California Dreamin'*. She asked that

I buy it for her. I listened to the song and noticed the beauty of Mama Cass's voice I'd missed all these years.

People occasionally ask me, "What are you?" I always say, "Mexican." This usually disturbs them; and interferes with their own foretold rendition of my identity. The choices on applications include "Black Hispanic" and "White non-Hispanic" and various other non sequiturs, given the reality of my birth. Such classification is even more absurd, assuming that's metaphysically possible, for my children, who are both Black and Mexican. Someone tried to clarify this for me: "You see, . . ." To which I replied, "No one has ever seen a Hispanic." He didn't catch my meaning. "Race," "ethnicity," or "ethniticity," as some, who apparently stammer to speak, take up time and space. Disagreement, disambiguation, and hair-splitting are all distractions from meaningful discourse, if we ever get to it. These hair-splitters distract from tangibility. Improvement. Concrete betterment. "Whites are now in the minority" assumes that Mexican, Puerto Rican, Cuban, Dominican, Chinese, Korean, Thai . . . are all interchangeable. (I suppose this same argument can be made for the Italo-German, a White guy.) One minority for another. I heard of a movement afoot: "I, too, am Harvard." The little I've heard overtly reminds me of our own "movement," which was exactly the same at Berkeley in the mid-1980s. My daughter, Black and Mexican, recalls a discussion among her classmates in middle school when a student told of a gang member wreaking havoc in a parking lot. Another classmate innocently asked, "Was he Black or Mexican?" My daughter sat quietly in her elite middle school, a new memory emerging from the oblivious early adolescent discourse. I don't know how long she will remain quiet. Not long, I trust. During a high school history class, the teacher noted: "We are all immigrants from somewhere." He then went around the class inviting the students to tell from whence their family came. When he arrived at my daughter's desk, she clarified, innocently, "My Dad's people were already here. My Mom's people came from Africa on slave ships. They don't really use the word, 'immigrant.'" Such is the colorful discourse available with a diverse student body.

I live in a White and Chinese neighborhood not far from Los Angeles. Indians, too, live here. Taiwanese, Korean, Pakistani, and others. We don't know any Mexicans near us. We are friends with the Black family here. Our children are classmates at the private college prep high school. I take our youngest daughter, an elementary school student, to the Debbie Allen Dance Academy in Los Angeles on Saturday mornings. DADA occupies a defunct Marie Callender's restaurant, I believe. DADA is across the parking lot from the movie theater Magic Johnson founded on Crenshaw Blvd. I heard that he sold it when he became part-owner of the Los Angeles Dodgers. (I don't earnestly keep up with these purchases and sales.) My daughter starts with tap, then African, then ballet, then hip hop. Four hours for me to spend nearby while I wait. I went to Magic's Starbuck's. I think it's gone by now. I had some emails to check, some chapters to edit, this chapter to write. People play chess at a table next to me. I watch two chess players, one White, one Black, start with rapid-fire moves initially. This reminds me of the carefree time when I learned to play chess during fourth grade. I could beat everyone in the school by the fifth grade, except for the sixth grader who'd taught me to play. The Black and White players slow after the flurry of opening moves, contemplating further choices—immediate, and ones to come soon afterward. Pensive. In Magic's Starbuck's were Black, White, a lesser number of Mexicans, and Central Americans. A Muslim family. A White young woman talks to a middle-aged Black man. I cannot tell if they already know each other or have just met. I think they know each other. A Japanese man talks with a Black couple. I don't know what anyone is talking about. I cannot hear. Through my headphones, I listen to "Jig-A-Jug," a piece on Joshua Redman's recorded collection, *Sprit of the Moment — Live*. In the end, the chess players stare at the black and white pieces, comtemplating the dearth of choices. I stop watching by then. I don't know who wins. I listen to "My One and Only Love."

I sat on a panel at a medical conference with two colleagues. I was there to talk about our previous book that invites the audience, with Aristotle's section on forensic discourse in mind, to evaluate health disparities differently, better than they are heretofore evaluated in standard medical journals. (I'd planned to address would-be solutions in a subsequent book.) One of us, a Chinese healthcare executive, started the discussion with a set of slides about healthcare in San Francisco's Chinatown. A slide with population data from Integrated Public Use Microdata Series 2006-2010 noted that Asian income, nationwide, is at 93% of White income. African Americans and Latinos are at 57% and 49%, respectively. These data, that certainly can be challenged, nevertheless struck me as peculiar when looking at Chinese people in San Francisco, specifically. That is, the income comparison for Chinese people in Chinatown is 47%, down there with us. It's easy enough to understand health disparities between Whites and Chinese people in Chinatown, as compared with Chinese people in, say, my neighborhood, when income disparities are conflated. So the lecture went. I then started speaking about the chapters in my last book. Before I could get very far, a man in the audience aggressively interrupted my speech and asked what solutions, if any, have been effective at decreasing the difference in health outcomes between the races. Another panelist addressed this question with a small example. More audience members joined the "discussion." We were never able to return to the arc of the *forensic* narrative that is necessary before we turn our attention to would-be solutions based on this evaluation.

Sometimes easy instrumental music plays overhead. I'd rather John Coltrane.

A Black guest on a news channel one blurred Sunday morning said to the newscaster about race in America, "We need to have an 'uncomfortable conversation' about race." I wasn't able to decipher to whom he was really speaking. Certainly not the newscaster. It's as if he were talking to the air. Who is this "we" he intends? Who would be uncomfortable? Why would "comfort" even be a variable worthy of stifling the "conversation"? The discomfort isn't nearly as bad as the outcomes of silence. I talk about race every day. It's not at all uncomfortable. In fact, I enjoy it. I call my friends from college and medical school and talk about race. I talk about race to Filipino, Chinese, Black, Mexican, Vietnamese, Indian, and White people, among others. I talk about race with old adults, forty or eighty years old, medical students, college students, teenagers, and my own children, who are in high, middle, and elementary school. I said to my youngest daughter that she looks like my eldest daughter. The youngest, who had studied tertiary colors in early elementary school by then, said, "No I don't. She's white. I'm brown." I don't get distracted when I talk about race—not when someone tries mightily to invoke class, socioeconomic status, gender, sexual orientation. We find ourselves very quickly talking about poor Whites in an Appalachia holler. We talk about "the system." About where money should be spent. About public education. About the children! About how race "should" be taught in medical school. (No one is good at identifying which current medical school lessons should be deleted in place of lessons on race; neither is anyone able to identify the race curriculum, much less the teachers. Nor are they able to articulate to what end these phantom lessons would lead.) In another news story, maybe a different Sunday, a California wildfire reached a neighborhood. Through the smoke, with no one in sight, a woman crawled down her driveway during the rapid fire burning through her neighborhood. She shouted out to anyone who might be in range to hear her. She shouted to the air: "Hey. I'm here. I'm alive."

5

Revoltist

A rhetoric professor, Rick Rigsby, Ph.D., who is also an ordained preacher, called me a revoltist. What did I say that made him call me this? In a Black preacher's crescendo, he preached: "Revoltist is a mindset. Some got it, some ain't. A revoltist is not *what* you do, but is the essence of *who* you are—your rebellious state of being. It's something that cannot be quantified with mere examples, or explained in the hope that others understand. Miles didn't give a damn whether you understood or not! The simple truth is, your essence embodies the denotative definition of the term, 'revolt': *To, in some manner or another, break away from constituted authority.* Why minimize the definition with passive examples in order to appease sensibilities? In other words, hit with blunt force. Jesus was a revoltist. Martin Luther King was a revoltist. Malcolm X was a revoltist. You don't get change without revoltists. I'm not a revoltist. I'm more of an assimilationist. People like me. But you go against the grain. The rest of us need you."

This sermon went on for a while. Because I couldn't interrupt the professor-preacher once he got on a roll, I had to let him finish, and then said, "You know, all those people got killed."

"I was hoping you didn't notice that. Give me a couple of weeks to get back to you."

I still haven't heard back from Rigsby about the deaths of these revoltists.

Why does the preacher need a revoltist? What good can come from a revoltist? "You don't get change . . ." connotes that change, itself, is vital, in order, prescribed.

I didn't try hard to figure out why he chose Jesus, Martin, and Malcolm in his oratory because he's a religious rhetor, and I figured these were stock samples of an elegant point about social healing he wanted to make directly to me. Jesus, the son of God, as it were, healed the sick with miracles. Martin stood in disobedience to injustice. Malcolm ignited minds.

I don't recall the first time I heard of Malcolm X, or the first time I heard one of his speeches. I do recall when I became conscious of X. While rummaging through the library at UC Berkeley as an undergraduate student I stumbled upon a VHS recording of a 1963 Malcolm X interview with a White political science professor and a Black graduate student. Amid the swirl of questions, affronts, and clarifications, Malcolm X began to talk about

Black people who had been officially documented as three-fifths of a human being by saying,

> "The Constitution was written *by* Whites for the benefit *of* Whites. It was never written for the benefit of Blacks. When you read the Constitution, I think in Article 1, Section 2, or Section 1, Article 1 . . . one of the two . . . it's in the Constitution. It classifies Black people as three-fifths of a man. *Three-fifths* of a man. Sub-human. Less than a human being. It relegates us as cattle, hogs, chickens, cows. A commodity that could be bought and sold at the will of the master."

The graduate student followed up with a question about a favorability poll. Before Malcolm X responded, he noted from a copy of the Constitution in a stack of references in his lap that included some of James Baldwin's writings related to recent church bombings, among other citations, which he referenced throughout the interview,

> "That statement I just made concerning the Constitution was Article 1, Section 2 in the Constitution where it classifies us as chattel."

Aside from Malcolm's majestic oratory, he dazzled me, a young college student, with the practice of carrying a reference section, rested on his lap, as he defended his ideas. I got lost in trying to find examples and hints of what Rigsby saw in me that prompted him to call me a revoltist. A 55-year-old defiant teenager, to be sure. Some might fruitlessly urge me to grow up.

Of course, Malcolm was wrong. Slaves were considered zero-fifths, which is how they were owned, and omitted, entirely, from enjoying the freedoms the U.S. Constitution addresses. The three-fifths was related to White male representation and collecting taxes from White slave owners.

What Rigsby is saying about Miles Davis is that he didn't "break the rules" as much as he didn't recognize their authority.

Another friend, a medieval English scholar with a concentration in linguistics, had read a couple of my early newspaper articles before we met, and said at our first dinner, "What I like about you is that you write against the grain. You don't follow the rules."

I said, "You got rules?"

The medieval English scholar blurted a guttaral laugh.

Any teacher of mine, beginning in the third grade, would say the same about me. I am naturally skeptical. It's God-given. Can't teach my disregard for authority. Got to be born with it. I start off disagreeing with someone telling me something. It's only after some serious, heavy, ad-hominecious debate that I might agree with him. But he will necessarily feel exhausted. I'd be invigorated. One colleague said to me after a business meeting, "I feel like I just had a cardio workout after a meeting with you." He was out of breath. I was rested.

I read something in the second book of personal essays written by Richard Rodriguez, *Days of Obligation: An Argument with my Mexican Father*: "*VETE PERO NO ME OLVIDES.*" This instruction was an unknown speaker addressing an unknown audience with antiquity at stake. The instruction, per se, didn't inspire me. I mean, I didn't emigrate from Mexico. When working on an essay a few years ago, for example, I asked my mother where my grandmother was born. My mother stared upward, into the distance, and, after some thought, said, "On the east side. In a house!" I was thinking, *Where on earth?* and estimating somewhere in Mexico, not somewhere in Stockton. My mother, too, was thinking, *Where on earth?* She considered Stockton the whole world. I stood corrected. The unknown speaker urging humanity not to forget as he left Mexico for California evoked in me an unsuspected vague melancholia I had never realized.

I don't write to say to an unknown audience that I am here. That they should not forget me. Not to a future that might be concerned with antiquity. But what can I do that will push against arc of history and bend the present so that we are not extinguished now, never mind whether we are forgotten in the future?

I had never looked to literature, or any other art, beyond its intrinsic beauty until after I finished medical school. I began playing the trumpet during a fourth-grade chance, and then met my genetic father, a jazz trumpeter, who offered me a first trumpet lesson in his mother's (my grandmother's?) house. I was instantly talented and ended up ascending to First Chair of the Advanced Symphonic Band in middle school. However, I didn't consider music as art when arranging my embouchure, practicing the scales, or playing First Chair. Rather, it was, to me, simply a class I took where I played the trumpet. Our music teacher, later in the year, invited this class of middle school musicians to the nearby junior college to hear an old flautist play with the symphony. I was the only student from my class who showed up. I didn't see my teacher, so I found a seat alone, near strangers who were at least five or six times my age. I listened to the beautiful sound and silently became aware that I enjoyed this music, which was starkly different from what I played in class or listened to on the radio at home, and thought, *This is good.*

I lived the rest of my Stockton adolescence silently appreciating intermittent instances of beauty, though not altogether consciously, where I inadvertently found them. I might have watched a movie and whispered to myself, *I like this*. I was moved by Shakespeare's *The Taming of the Shrew* the in the twelfth grade, and, later that year, found *Othello's* Iago breathtaking. I appreciated *Alvin Ailey* ballet dancers who performed at Zellerbach Theater on campus when I was at Berkeley. I discovered Sarah Vaughan and Miles Davis during medical school. I watched a PBS show, *Spirituals in Concert*, featuring opera singers Kathleen Battle and Jessye Norman, and flautist Hubert Laws. I read Latin American and Russian literature during my training in pediatrics: Gabriel García Márquez, Jorge Luis Borges, Octavio Paz, Juan Rulfo, Fyodor Dostoyevsky, Nikolai Gogol. Still later, I grew into the personal capacity to find literary inspiration in bebop's Thelonious Monk. Van Gogh, Vermeer, Dvořák. In fact, I'm listening to Rachmaninov: Piano Concerto #2 In C Minor, Op. 18 - 1. Moderato as I type these sentences.

Toni Morrison noted that art for art's sake is a relatively new idea— only about 150 years old. Something like that. "Art ought to *do* something." Of course, in my line of work as a pediatrician, effervescent passages about antiquity or a far-off future, if there is one, cannot exist. There are binary clinical demands impervious to, and impatient with, purple prose, and jazzprose, in medicine. "What is the tangible solution to race in America?" my suffering friend asks, trying to move me from the ethereal to the corporeal.

We pour another drink of Scotch and tell some more stories.

Another friend of mine, a social science professor, wrote an analysis of inequality in medicine based on race, but did not suggest any concrete solutions. I asked him about this? He said, "I'm a professor. I live to ask questions. Someone else would need to provide the answers."

We laugh.

Increased death rate, excess limb amputations, kidney failure, diabetic blindness, undiagnosed cancer, unchecked high blood pressure, the continued truth that Black infant mortality is over twice that of White infant mortality, which has not decreased in the recent few decades despite medical progress.

I attended a noon lecture at an elite medical school some years ago. The speakers talked about a race-specific drug to treat heart failure. There was some discussion about hypertension among Black people, how the doctors might determine whether someone is Black, whether the "data" is self-reported, or whether the registration clerk simply assigns the patient's race by looking at his physical features from across the registration counter, and social v.

biological definitions of race. By the end of this tiresome elite medical conference I raised my hand and said, "I'm just a pediatrician, but I can't help but wonder if someone had addressed this Black man's high blood pressure that resulted in his congestive heart failure a couple of decades earlier, wouldn't any talk about his race, and whether this or that medicine is best, be superfluous?"

The leader of the noon conference, my friend, looked at me and said, "You party pooper."

I mentioned this episode in an exchange of a few letters with renowned Professor of History at Columbia University, Barbara Fields, that prompted her response to me about my question at the elite medical school conference: "We need more party poopers."

My initial article on race and medicine, "The Misuse of Race in Medical Diagnoses," published in *The Chronicle of Higher Education*, argued against the required template to include the patient's race at the very beginning of a medical presentation, either verbal or written. I did not initially think such an article was worthy of publication. My best man, a rhetorician, said, "But you're going against a mainstay of medical school teaching that *all* medical students have been taught for the last hundred years. And you're correct. You ought to publish this."

It was only after I'd published that first article on race and medicine that I looked further into the topic.

Because I'd always been interested in race, sociology, Ethnic Studies, and such, I continued to read novels and social science articles in these areas as a nostalgic effort reminding me of the kind of intellectual life I might have led were it not for medical school. The first lecture I recall on this topic was in a conference room in the basement of a hospital next to the cafeteria: "Cultural Competence." I had not yet heard that term, and could not know what it meant. Naturally, it sounded important. The speaker highlighted people from around the world, their languages, their food, their style of dress, and other social realities that reminded me of my high school cultural anthropology class. I was disappointed that there was no substance to the talk. No urgency that I understood in Richard Wright's novels, in James Baldwin's personal essays, in Malcolm X's speeches.

I attended other such lectures in medical circles. I started looking for articles about race, but found that they were about health disparities, and chronicled decades of inequalities in healthcare service and in physical health outcomes. One article, then another—each chronicling the disparities between races. I eventually understood that analogous disparities based on race could easily be seen in education, business, law enforcement, and the other American institutions. However, I didn't think that the habit of chronicling how bad things are for darker people would be useful. We've already gotten all we're going to get originating in guilt. And in reality. There is a void between the analysis of such chronicles and the invention of solutions based on these analyses. I found a contagion of people splitting the hairs of health disparities; and there was a runaway movement toward the standard thinking—minorities need translators, they need black and brown doctors, they need insurance cards—an inertia that would not stop on its own. But Black people speak English. Mexicans speak English. People on Medicaid have insurance. I could see that the bandwagon would not lead to the invention of missing humanity with respect to race even if academics got tenure for their publications, got paid for their speeches, got recognized for their expertise.

There exists a passive, perennial need to revolt. The tried and true standard approaches to addressing health outcomes disparities based on race—workforce diversity, cultural competence, health insurance, language translation—while important, seem directed at correcting some deficiency of the patients. If only they spoke English, if only they were insured, if only they were White. But insured, English-speaking White people are suffering in American medicine. This is nightly news. There's nothing wrong with speaking Spanish, with being Cambodian. What good is a cheap health insurance card in a man's wallet if there are no doctors available—and willing!—to see him?

These would-be solutions are approaches to manage the deficiencies in patients; not deficiencies in medicine, in society, that continue, retrigger, and sustain centuries-old disparities. It's an old, tired statement that the health outcomes in the United States are far beneath the outcomes of other countries, made to sound worse because the United States pays far more for these poor outcomes when compared with other countries. This argument is not about money, per se, of course, because if we paid less and had poor outcomes, we should not be so satisfied. And if we had superior outcomes, the price would still be too high. Then, the argument is: treat minorities as badly as you treat Whites, and we'll call that progress. But as Malcolm X noted when interviewed about progress once he was able to speak publicly after he'd been silenced for his "chickens have come home to roost" comment, "If you stick a knife in my back nine inches and pull it out six inches, there's no progress. If you pull it all the way out that's not progress. Progress is healing the wound that the blow made. And they haven't even pulled the knife out, much less heal the wound. They won't even admit the knife is there." Malcolm X understood that progress was not forthcoming.

What is the hope of a revoltist? Tangible change? Better thinking? To challenge and refine heretofore approaches that could be replaced, or supplemented, with better ones? Like August Wilson described himself, I was a race guy as a Berkeley undergraduate student before heading to medical school. I'm accustomed to incisive discussions about the entrenched habits that cause, and maintain, disparities. A frail plea to appreciate the other, to get me a language translator, is preordained to fail. I appreciate blues singer Bessie Smith's sensibility, "No matter how cruel he may be, it won't be you. And if he beats me, and breaks my heart, it won't be you." She understands that there is no end to the trauma in sight. Even if she is not hopeful, she perseveres. Bessie Smith revolts.

Part Two

Barriers and Old Ideas

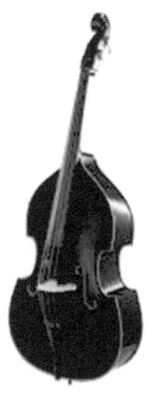

6

Dismantling

The Boulé is a fraternity of educated elite Black men. I initially heard of this group in the 1980s when I was a pre-medical student at Berkeley. I'd met a family of doctors who took me in when they heard I might want to become a pediatrician and work in my distressed neighborhood in south Stockton. The family appreciated my early dedication and decided to take me, a poor Mexican pre-medical student, with them to the Asilomar Conference Grounds along the California central coast to the Boulé.

As a routine during the weekend retreat I sat around with Supreme Court of California Associate Justice Allen B. Broussard, the University of California Vice President for Health Affairs, the recent president of the National Bar Association, professors from nearby universities, and physi- cians who worked in Oakland. The president of the Boulé that year led retreat discussions about how these esteemed Black men would work in keeping with their mission to help poor Black people.

I recently chatted with one of the medical school professors, retired by now, who noted that an early draft of this chapter about these Black pioneers brought back fond memories for him. "The setting was perfect and the atmosphere was highly conducive to 'getting to know the best of one another'—one of our Boulé mantras. As time moves on, our ranks are, of course, thinning (I will be 83 in August), but the memories generated during those years are priceless. And sustaining."

A group of Black doctors descended into Oakland, California in the 1960s. Most had completed undergraduate studies at Black colleges and universities, and then graduated from one of the Black medical schools. One of these doctors, originally from Charleston, South Carolina, graduated from Virginia State College for Negroes, and then Meharry Medical College in Nashville, Tennessee. The state of South Carolina paid for his Tennessee medical education because he was not legally allowed to attend a White medical school in South Carolina. His influential classmates and colleagues practiced medicine in and around Oakland where they took care of primarily poor Black people for the rest of their careers.

I thought about becoming a pediatrician during my freshman year as an undergraduate student at Berkeley. My idea was to return to nearby Stockton, a miserable city, as published in recent surveys, and work across the street from my high school with my own pediatrician, who had gone to medical school with some of the Black doctors in Oakland. Within the first few weeks of college I went on a hospital tour with four other premedical students—each of us either Black or Mexican—where I was able to talk directly with a doctor about medical school. None of us had ever talked with a doctor about our ambitions. The touring pediatrician walked us around the hospital, pointed things out, and gently dismantled any barriers between medicine and us. By the end of the robust tour, I had no sense of what it might mean to be a doctor. The pediatric resident asked if we had any further questions. I raised my hand and asked a question in the most sophisticated way I was able: "What happens when poor children come to the ER?"

This is still a good question today, even if I can pose it in finer language.

An awesome unreality for me, I went to medical school and became a pediatrician. I am repeatedly questioned about my own "success" as a poor Mexican from Stockton with three generations of men in prison, and my genetic father and two of my uncles, all who were to die from respective overdoses of heroin in the coming few years, representing my possibilities in life. I'm endlessly asked about my own *survival* as if I were hunted game whose conclusion was foretold by my family history of early violent deaths, even through today. I recently quipped to a national medical figure that all of my uncles and my eldest cousin were in prison during my adolescence, a time where I might have been most vulnerable to their influence: "I suppose I have the State of California penitentiary system to thank."

Perhaps this wasn't really a playful grace note.

I ultimately became the "adopted" son of this Black family of doctors and attended birthday parties, local medical meetings, national medical conventions, and family reunions. I met new "cousins," and generally belonged on the family's inside.

The National Medical Association is an organization that began in the late 1800s when Black doctors were disallowed by the American Medical Association, and can loosely, and incorrectly, be described as the Black version of the AMA. I tagged along with the rest of the family to the NMA Convention and went to the president's installation ceremony. As one of the Black doctors from Oakland awaited his acceptance speech, he called me to his hotel room. "I want you to go around to all of my brothers and sisters in the hotel and ask them for something of theirs that I can wear when I'm onstage giving my acceptance speech." I didn't understand what was happening, but dutifully found each sibling, four older and four younger, and asked for an article that their middle brother, the family's master negotiator as the middle child of nine children, might wear.

Some ask me questions, which I could not answer. Others simply understood their brother and gave me cuff links, a handkerchief, an undershirt, a pin. I gave the President-elect his siblings' articles as he dressed for his acceptance speech. I would recount this story at his funeral many years later at the Church by the Side of the Road where I wore a blue tie he had given me one evening when he took me to a medical meeting. I negotiated the tie from him and wore it for years, and thought it would be nice to wear in the pulpit when I spoke at his funeral service.

I spent the last month of medical school as a student in a pediatrician's office in Oakland who was a part of this group of Black doctors. The pediatrician had completed his undergraduate degree at Fisk, a Black university in Nashville, where he was a member of the famous Jubilee Singers. He then went to Meharry Medical College, graduated, and moved out west to Oakland to set up his pediatrics practice. I'd arranged to spend the last month of medical school in his office because I thought I could learn what I did not learn in medical school en route to a career in a pediatrics practice like his.

He was sixty-one years old by then. He had a tennis court in his backyard and invited me to play a match. Young, fit, eager, I accepted the sixty-one-year-old's challenge and quickly began my braggadocio. He let me finish, and then noted that I'd forgotten the most important part, and pointed to his temple: "The mind." We drove to his house and played a set of tennis. I won the set in a vicious tiebreaker, and hobbled to the chair, finished for the day.

The sixty-one-year-old pediatrician clarified that this was two out of three sets, and urged me to get back on the court. "Boy, you better get up."

Debilitated and scared, I agreed.

6-6. At the beginning of the second set tiebreaker, I understood that I had better win this second set because I would be wholly unable to play a third set, would forfeit, and would have to contend with his braggadocio for the duration of my rotation as a medical student in his office.

I won the second tiebreaker. We went into the house where one of the older doctors waited for us in the air-conditioned living room. He asked who won. The old pediatrician said, "The jackrabbit—but barely."

I learned the greatest lesson of my medical education during the next week in his office. I saw a poor baby brought in by his mother at the end of the afternoon. I asked her about the baby, but didn't get much clinical information to help me. I examined the baby, but didn't understand what I found. I asked the mother to hold her baby while I went to get the pediatrician. She was relieved, I suppose, because she had brought her baby to see him, and not me. When he arrived at the exam room doorway, he stood there and looked inside. He turned to me and, in a voice louder than required, said, "Look at this child! He looks miserable. I want you to remember this look."

We drove the baby, the mother, and the other children to the nearby hospital because asking her to take them on the bus would have been too much to ask.

Other Black doctors worked like this in Oakland. I met with them through the years, saw them at conventions, birthday parties, scattered university lectures. These men inspired my college classmates and me, and stood among us prepared to help guide our careers in ways that would replace theirs someday.

One of the doctors, for example, formed an alliance between the Black physicians and the Black preachers of Oakland because he understood that even if Black people didn't see their doctors during the week, they would see their preachers at church on Sundays. The collective of Black physicians hosted healthcare clinics after church, evening meetings to strategize how they might generally help Black people in and around Oakland, and structured a blood pressure screening extravaganza that included medical students from Stanford, the University of California at San Francisco, and the University of California at Berkeley, nurses from the pews, and the Black doctors, themselves, in a coordinated strike timed to coincide with the end of the respective Bay Area Black church services.

Concerned about the high rate and aggressive nature of prostate cancer among Black men, and their general reluctance to get prostate exams, a Black urologist enlisted some of the professional baseball players of the Oakland A's to help him campaign among Black men to encourage them to seek this particular medical care.

When the first one of these Black doctors died, the others thought that someone should write a history of what they achieved in Oakland. Because I'd written some medical articles by then, one of them thought I should work on this project. He and I went to talk with the widow. He told me that her husband was a surgeon in an integrated military company during the Korean War. The widow offered a corrective: "*He* integrated the company."

I spoke with one of the other Black doctors about this untold history when we met at a medical event at the Oakland Convention Center. He noted that this was not a good idea because "The entire history has to be written. Someone will have to explain the times, what was going on, and how we all fit into that time." He thought that simple recounts of the events would be anemic versions of a considerable American reality, and would ultimately fail.

I couldn't help but agree and stopped working on the project. As more of the Black doctors died, I'd forgotten about the hunger for this history. No one encouraged me further to write about the era of these Black doctors. In fact, I recently met a young Black doctor who noted that most of his contemporaries aren't even members of the NMA, but have formed a remote, electronic organization for young Black doctors.

Though I am not Black, I do think about this decrescendo in healthcare for poor Black people. My own goal was to return to my home in Stockton and work in my pediatrician's office across the street from my high school. In the end, I took my career into executive and administrative medicine, and out of my neighborhood. Paralyzed by enduring reality, perhaps I souled out.

I recently spoke with the Dean of Academic Affairs at a Midwestern medical school who showed me the class picture and pointed to the Black students who were about to graduate: interventional radiology, dermatology, ENT, etc. Only one of the twelve graduating seniors planned a career in primary care medicine. Certainly, Black people need these subspecialists. And certainly, these Black subspecialists will take care of people who are not Black. However, there exists a dearth of day-to-day doctors in Black neighborhoods. In Mexican neighborhoods. Who will teach a medical student to remember a miserable Black child's face?

These doctors are dying out. Of course, some students return. Some of these doctors' children went to medical school and returned, my classmate from Berkeley, and others have returned. But this arc is not sustained. It's not nurtured enough.

I gave a speech at Berkeley's School of Public Health a couple of years ago and asked a Nigerian graduate student where all the Black people were. She said, "They're gone." I told her about my time at Berkeley in the 1980s. Her face lit up and she said, "We heard about those days!"

As I've discussed my own writings about health outcomes disparities, my well-meaning friends worry about a book that doesn't offer concrete answers. Some are concerned that non-linear, "impressionistic" writing might not be applicable for medical concepts that require linear, if not concrete, writing. To be sure, as a doctor trained in pediatric emergency medicine where I routinely took helicopters and Learjets to pick up dying babies and return them to university hospitals, I am most definitely able to think and communicate with clarity and linearity. There's no room for quirky allegories when a baby might die in the coming seconds.

These chapters are not recipes that can be deployed like, say, a recipe for oatmeal cookies, that the reader will be able to lift, employ in some desperate neighborhood, and end up with equal health outcomes for Black or Mexican people, and a batch of oatmeal cookies. Rather, as such concretized ideas are considered for Oakland or Detroit or Chicago or Stockton or New Orleans or Houston or Atlanta or Los Angeles or D.C., a sensibility and a history with which would-be solutions should be considered is in order.

That is, like Dorothy in *The Wiz*, we already know the solution to health disparities. The Oakland doctors provided them in a Sisyphean effort in the last half of the twentieth century. They provided exemplary healthcare to Black people for a generation—a reification that could still work, but is fading as the old doctors die. Their work could be a template for now. But these efforts, like the ones in the previous century, have been dismantled over the last couple of decades. Then asking a question about what *can* tangibly be done now about health outcomes disparities is not a genuine question. There is some other question that's more to the point: What *will* we do about the dismantling? Of course, this "we" is its own question: Who is this "we"? And will we remember the time before the dismantling? This is not a medical question; but a human one.

Medicine is different now. Confederacy states don't pay tuition for Black students disallowed at home. *De jure* segregation, generally, is gone, even if it generally remains, *de facto*. Millennial students, no matter their color, might imagine balance between life and work, and might also imagine geometrically rising incomes in the face of titanic debt and an explosive cost of living. The life of a primary care physician, let alone one in solo practice, is an unreality when compared with the nostalgic, flowery San Francisco Bay city of Oakland of the 1960s. Which doctor will type "M-I-S-E-R-A-B-L-E" in an Electronic Medical Record if she's not able to find it in a drop-down list or as a predetermined smart phrase? Young doctors might prefer a health system like Kaiser, or another employed-physician group, for example, as a safe landing strip where Paid Time Off and absolute M-F working hours are plainly typed into the employment contract. The style of medicine in Oakland of a few decades ago paid attention to poor Black people. That style was not sustained. Now, it seems that some hybrid approach that recalls the mission to work there, in Oakland, on purpose, is in order, and ought to be folded into modernity. This cannot be a recipe; but can be an idea, nevertheless.

James Baldwin said, "I can't be a pessimist, because I am still alive." The Black doctors of Oakland took me in. They concretized their pre-medical school idea to take care of Black people there, where no one else would. Such tangible efforts, even amidst any oratory flurry, are required to address disparities, if we are to be optimistic. If we are still alive.

7

Where's Barrington?

A man from Ghana told me that "*Obroni*" means "White man" in his language. He left home a long time ago to attend a university in New Jersey. He returns home for extended visits when he gets the chance. If he is away from Ghana for too long, he is called "*Obroni*" by his family and by his countrymen when they affectionately tease him upon his return. I laughed when he told me that he was called this after spending too much time in the United States. I tried to calculate how much was too much, but couldn't do the arithmetic. I don't know many Africans. I thought about the first time I'd ever considered a real African. This was a South African tennis player I would watch on TV from time to time when I was a child. I was a great tennis fan in the days before the recent ability to digitally record television shows. I recall watching the finals of, say, Wimbledon or the U.S. Open, and admiring the drop shot Bjorn Borg retrieved and then deftly located the tennis ball diagonally, imperceptibly over the net where his opponent had no chance to reach the ball sensationally now back on his side of the court. I could not pause the match in those days, but found the television commercials useful chances to get a snack or a cold drink during the hot summer adolescent days of Stockton. Of course, now I can fast forward right through the commercials without watching them; and I can pause the match whenever I please. I can watch more, and more efficient, tennis, including the early rounds, such that I can now appreciate players who might not have made it to the televised finals weekends of my youth. I recall being perplexed as a child when watching a South African tennis player who was white. I had not yet gone to college at Berkeley where we were to protest the university's investment in South Africa when I learned about its policy of apartheid. The protest lectures on Sproul Plaza, in front of Sather Gate, the university's *de facto* insignia, recalled for us Berkeley undergraduates: slavery, Dred Scott, Jim Crow, Ida B. Wells, Fannie Lou Hamer, and the others, right up through to the urgent present of those past days. Until then I had considered that Africans were black, and not white. In fact, I still struggle against my primitive understanding, and am still startled when I see an African who is not black. Of course, I understand that they exist. But my mental sketch, my primordial template, the prototype in my mind when I think of an

Where's Barrington?

African includes my Nigerian friends, my Ghanaian friends, and not at all my children, for example, who seem to me both Black and Mexican—children from me and my wife, whose people were slaves in Mississippi before their trudge to Chicago, and then onward west, to Los Angeles. Though I occasionally find myself passively reminding these children of ours that they are Mexican, that they are Black, that they are not White, I don't think they listen to me on this topic. They retreat to their classmates: Indian, Korean, Chinese, Taiwanese, White.

The editor of a prestigious medical journal invited a medical school Dean of Admissions to write an article about the difference between "African American" applicants and "African" applicants. This is a barbed dare with the distinct possibility, if not intent, to divide and conquer [emphasis on "conquer"] by pitting descendants of slaves against recent immigrants from Africa who appear congruous, but live distinct lineages when compared with Black people in the United States, and are, themselves, varied people from the continent of Africa, with its fifty-four countries, give or take. Writing such an article risks pitting brother against brother, should anyone fall for such duplicitous academic bait.

The risk here is to conflate two pivotal variables when considering medical education: so-called "diversity" and the intent of late-20th century pushes to include racial minorities—namely Black, Puerto Rican, Mexican American, and Native American—in medical schools because they, more than anyone else, the data routinely show, will likely return to their own cities and neighborhoods and help their poor people.

But if the Spanish Basque can pass for "Hispanic," and the school can claim an African, these days, instead of a Black young man from Oakland or Chicago or Atlanta, as was the intent of such American academic integration, then so-called "diversity" is achieved. (I'm aware that there are actual Africans in those cities. But I'm not talking about them.) I looked at an early draft of the dean's article en route to submission to the prestigious journal and tried to help. I immediately noticed that he used the term "African American" to mean Black people, like him, whose people were slaves in the arc of American history. The clunky linguistics worsened when trying to isolate people in the United States who recently emigrated from Africa to attend graduate school, let's say. I read further, and had practical questions. I became honestly confused, and asked, "When you say 'African,' do you mean people from Tunisia? Algeria? Morocco? That white-skinned tennis player from my childhood?"

The medical school dean clarified, "I mean Sub-Saharan Africa."

Naturally, this did not clarify things for me. Is South Africa not below the Sahara? Are Nigerians so simply interchangeable with Congolese? Does an Angolan, with his legacy of Portuguese imperialism, live the nuances of his neighbor in Zambia, after his independence from Britain?

The reason for so-called diversity in academia, as I understand university websites and overt verbal claims, is so that the milieu of the classroom and the campus can be fortified for the benefit of White students. Minorities don't require such fortification of a diverse milieu. We are the diversity. This is not a criticism, but a corrective along the lines of when there is talk, and policy, about "Women and Minorities," which is a clandestine translation of "*White* Women and Minorities" because minority women would already be captured in the "Minorities" part of the insolent dyad. Diversity in academia, to be sure, can be understood as a good thing. It can also be understood as perfunctory, insincere, isolating.

The other component of so-called diversity in medical education is more corporeal than visual, virtual diversity that might foster a richer classroom discourse than could be expected without skin-deep, artificial diversity.

The Civil Rights exhortation was to invite minorities to medical school so that they might return to their desperate neighborhoods and deliver medical care, and not so that esteemed White students might enjoy colorful banter en route to their White adulthoods. Then, medical education insofar as it intersects with delivering medical care to underserved—and unserved!—neighborhoods, especially, *depends* upon medical school classrooms that include students already interested in working in these vast and growing areas of our country. More than wanting to work in these areas, in fact, what's predictive, according to Somnath Saha, MD, MPH, Professor of Medicine at Oregon Health and Sciences University, in his January/February 2008 *Health Affairs* article, "Race-Neutral Versus Race-Conscious Workforce Policy to Improve Access to Care," is that medical students who emerge from these neighborhoods are the most likely to return to work there, where they are sorely needed.

Or else, the Urban Health Program at the University of Illinois College of Medicine recognizes that those medical school applicants who are *already predisposed* to working in poor minority areas provide the most hope of delivering healthcare there. If the goal is to achieve a healthcare workforce that reflects the diversity of the United States, stated explicitly by the Association of American Medical Colleges, the American Medical Association, and the Institute of Medicine, as noted in the October 2006 U.S. Department of Health and Human services publication, "The Rationale for Diversity in the Health

Professions: A Review of the Evidence," can be believed as true, then this would-be truth could be coupled with the possibility that both diversity *and* direct healthcare delivery has a Venn diagram sweet spot found among minority students from these very communities.

The president of a local, inner-city chapter of the National Medical Association received a call from an African doctor working in Barrington. He told the president of an episode of racism, and wondered if the NMA could help. The local NMA president listened to the entire claim of suburban racism and then asked, "Where's Barrington? You should be here helping us take care of Black people in the city."

I asked a leader among physicians in Oakland about the dearth of Black doctors in places that need them most, which seems to be worsening as the elders from just a generation ago are retiring or dying without forthcoming reinforcements. He noted that legal segregation was no good; but that integration did not fulfill its promise. In fact, it didn't have a real chance before being rolled back.

A continuum is required.

I gave a lecture at a local medical school where I met some of the students devoted to working in a largely Mexican city in southern California when they complete their medical training. One of the Mexican students grew up in central California and then went to the University of California at Berkeley. On the next beat, as a Mexican who grew up in central California and then went to Berkeley, I said, "I know everything you know!" He laughed, and agreed. We became friends, met occasionally to discuss the rest of his medical education, and explored the possibilities for his next step: residency training. In the end, after I'd pushed him to consider what he plans for his career with poor Mexicans, and why, beyond the obvious self-portrait, he plans such a career, and why he chose pediatrics. I helped review his personal statement and offered suggestions about what he might write. I said, "You can't simply say that you grew up poor and Mexican and want to return to your community as a doctor to help because we all wrote that same thing thirty years ago. You'll need to write something better." I was only joking with the medical student, who ultimately procured a prestigious pediatrics residency, and is now on his way to a career in academic medicine as a pediatric cardiologist. I felt defeated, however, *because* we had written those same sentences in our personal statements to medical school and residency thirty years ago, just like the generations before us wrote, and are, nevertheless, still confronted with the dilapidated health outcomes such that current minority medical school applicants can include these same sentences, still applicable, in their hopeful prose.

I also reviewed the personal statement of an undergraduate student as she prepared her application to medical school. I changed some verbs from passive to active; moved one paragraph up, to the beginning; changed some adjectives; deleted a word here and there. I worry that poor minority applicants cannot afford—or, like me during this early stage, don't know to afford—tangible help, that works in concert with family and neighborhood encouragement, to finish medical education and training, to then come back home to help, where they are especially needed. Now, like before.

8

In Baltimore, Once

I met a nearby English professor during the brief time I worked as a medical school professor. I looked through the various departments on the university website to see who I might find to discuss literature, sociology, Ethnic Studies, or other topics I suspected real academics might discuss. Because I was a faculty member of the medical school where I worked clinically, and not scholarly, I thought I should find real academic colleagues with whom I might become friends. I searched the department websites and looked for people who worked in areas in which I was already interested, or else, in areas in which I should be interested. I'd only recently discovered Latin American literature by then, so I started there. I'd also longed for a chance to dust off my old undergraduate sociology discussions and Ethnic Studies theses. I found a few entries in the list of faculty in some of the pertinent departments. One professor, a Mexican, from what I could tell on the webpage posting, stood out as almost kindred. He had taken his Ph.D. at Stanford in Modern Thought and Literature, a sort of combination of sociology, philosophy, and English, I imagined. His area of specialty was American Literature, and his dissertation was on Richard Wright's work, I believe, which lured me closer as I contemplated what appeared to be dissonant doctoral scholarship by a Mexican.

We exchanged a few emails, then met for lunch near the university. This turned into a friendship where I suspect I benefited more from our talks about literature. I'd reached Latin American literature during my training in pediatrics, after having read Afro-American literature in college, to the point that I considered a Ph.D. in literature when someone told me that because I already have a "terminal degree" I didn't need a Ph.D. for what I had in mind. I could simply read and write what I wanted. I eventually understood that he didn't mean "terminal" the way we mean it in medicine, and agreed. I shamelessly asked unorthodox questions of my new English professor friend and haphazardly filled in the literary lessons I had not learned during my formal education leading up to medical school, or even during my informal education when I was on the loose reading Camus without guidance. The English professor was, however, unusually interested in the details of medical education, the practice of medicine, and in *how* to locate ordinary healthcare ideas into his academic scheme. Our conversations oscillated freely between Borges and cancer, Ellison and diabetes, Kafka and psychosis. I suppose the English professor benefited, too, from our friendship.

He told me of the resistance he received from the Black students who questioned his ethos when he arrived on campus to teach African American literature. Shortly, the students understood that he was qualified; and that their misplaced outrage could finally be downgraded to annoyance. He quickly found my interest in literature to be sincere, and invited me to audit his upcoming course: Faulkner and García Márquez.

Because I submitted to the seismic shift in *how* I understood the entire world after reading Gabriel García Márquez's *One Hundred Years of Solitude* on my own, long after I'd graduated from college, I was giddy at the chance to read this novel in a class with a professor—a chance to supplement my limited understanding, though seismic, of the greatest novel. I confessed to the English professor that I'd read William Faulkner's *Light in August* as an undergraduate student in college, but didn't remember it; and that I failed to finish *The Sound and the Fury* because I didn't understand the first chapter. He laughed, assured me that many don't understand that first chapter, if it can even be understood, and encouraged me to audit his class with even more resolve: "We're reading *Absalom, Absalom!* You'll like it. You'll get it."

We kept in touch through the years after I left the medical school faculty, chatting mostly about literary things, including my own publications, which started after I left academia. He remained interested in medicine, and admired my dedication to world literature in English, which included works from China, Japan, India, Nigeria, and elsewhere by then, however informal. We talked on the phone about presidential elections, race in academia, race in medicine, disparities based on race in the various social institutions, and wondered how we might work together. We appreciated our mutual ability to juxtapose disparate fields of study as we discussed this or that social question.

Race was the big one.

I was working out an idea for a collection of personal essays about health disparities and thought that a team of us—physicians and non-physicians—should contribute to the collection since I understood race in medicine to be a subset of race in America. He agreed to help me with the book, and contributed a chapter. He also helped me review other chapters written by the interdisciplinary group interested in writing personal essays on race and medicine: sociology, psychology, rhetoric, cardiology, vascular surgery, geriatrics, and so forth, including two medical school deans. In the end, we finished the collection and submitted it for publication at an academic press, where the manuscript was accepted.

This was all very exciting for me, a non-academic, though meant nothing along the lines of promotion and tenure, as it might for real academics. Still, I hoped to do some good, publish a book on race and medicine, and continue to work in medicine in ways that might incorporate my attention to humanities and social sciences.

The English professor mentioned that he belongs to some academic organizations analogous to the medical organizations to which I belong. As we finalized the edits of the personal essay collection, he suggested that we should submit a proposal to speak at an interdisciplinary academic conference where we might find an audience, or at least some compatriots, in this "field" of scholarship. He figured that a group with self-proclaimed interdisciplinarity as the crux of their scholarship would be a natural place for us to discuss our book about health disparities written in the personal essay form by physicians, medical school deans, and social science and humanities professors.

I looked at the conference submission guidelines and didn't understand the very words used to describe the conference, I confess. The guidelines appeared to be disciplinary, sanctioned social science jargon. I could not tell whether our interdisciplinary chapters on race and medicine would apply to such submission criteria, so I wrote to the conference organizer in plain prose to see if what we were up to was in keeping with that year's conference theme, which I could not decipher. She replied that our work was very much in keeping with the theme, and gave examples. I copied and pasted those examples into my submission, added a few medical details marking the human decay in medicine when comparing people from different races, and sent this hybrid to the selection committee.

Our roundtable panel was accepted.

Five of us flew to the convention in Baltimore. Two MDs, an MD, MBA, an MD, Ph.D., and a Ph.D. comprised our ragtag group.

En route to the session, as I gathered my thoughts about how I would introduce our speakers, I asked my friend, the MD, Ph.D., who was the Deputy Provost at an elite university, "Are you over just the medical school or the whole thing?" He said, "The whole thing. I just hired a poet and a physicist last week." That's all I needed to complete my thoughts about what I'd say in the form of our introduction prior to our presentation.

During the English professor's introduction, which was scheduled to be extremely brief, he mentioned the "medical industrial complex," a phrase I'd never heard physicians use. In fact, until that very moment, I'd never even heard of it. The cardiologist among us later explained this to me in both medical and military terms. I still didn't get it.

Before I could further our introductions, a professor in the audience raised a question about our qualifications. He noted that we were listed in the conference brochure as "Independent Scholars," but worked for health insurance companies. The cardiologist tried to smooth things over and quipped, "I work for Kaiser. I'm neither independent nor a scholar. You'll need to talk to whoever created the conference brochure."

Other professors in the audience chimed in and continued the affront before I could get through the introductions. One sociologist, I think she was, offered: "What you're saying is nothing new. It's twenty-five years old." She then listed some disciplinary books and articles and deduced that we had not even bothered to read them. Others in the scholarly mob seemed to agree, and, in a final thump, accused us of being physicians.

Because this was not a medical conference, but a conference of professors who, from what I could tell, worked in mostly social science and humanities spheres—which is why we thought this would be the perfect interdisciplinary venue for physicians looking to collaborate with these spheres as we considered health disparities based on race—I did not know how I should respond to the academic pummeling. As physicians, of course, it's easy for us to combat each other now that we've wrestled with surgeons during medical school and residency. We've all scrapped with a consultant with whom we disagreed. Who among us has not warded off an irate, incorrect attending physician trying to "teach" us some obscure clinical point? But *how* to tussle with social science and humanities hostilities, I admit, caught me off of my natural, eternal guard. I felt like the prostitute protagonist in *Pretty Woman* who was impotent when confronted with a would-be John at a polo match, and noted that she could handle a guy like that if she were in her own clothes on Hollywood Boulevard. She'd be prepared.

I turned to the Deputy Provost, the MD, Ph.D., whom I hadn't yet had the chance to introduce, and asked him if we should start taking questions before we've even finished our introductions, if we should finish our introductions, give our talks, and *then* take questions, or just let things go on in this scholarly morass. He leaned back in his chair, cool, which was a starkly different rhetorical and physical stance than the rest of us took, and said, "Let her finish."

When things died down, he said, "Not only have I read all of the things you just listed, I wrote some of them." He then went on to defend the panel, our role at the conference, and the importance of an interdisciplinary approach to the centuries-laden health disparities between the races in America.

The discussion devolved. Though I failed at leading this unruly discourse, I desperately tried to maintain some modicum of professionalism because we physicians were guests at the social science and humanities academic conference. Mercifully, time ran out, and the session ended.

We never went back.

I wondered if my syllogism was wrong: Race in medicine is a subset of race in America. Addressing race requires insight from various academic fields. Interdisciplinarity is required to address health disparities based on race.

Crossing disciplinary jargons is hazardous, I found. While I did not understand the very words, let alone the combination of words, used in even the conference submission guidelines, I don't suppose the sociologist, for example, could follow the shorthand in what I might say to the pediatric cardiologist: "The kid's fussy." This is not the colloquial fussiness that anyone can understand, but a distinct and key term that speaks to a pediatric cardiologist and must be included in his evaluation of a dying baby along with the results of other cardiac studies. What would we look like if we were to chastise a sociologist, let's say, for not having understood, or even bothered to read, my article on inpatient v. outpatient UPPP in the *Journal of Otolaryngology – Head & Neck Surgery*?

How can we concretize would-be solutions to health disparities if the various disciplines even wanted to collaborate because they agreed that my syllogism is not wrong? Whether we would understand each other, which would be subsequent to wanting to talk, is a separate question. That is, in order to concretize our ideas about would-be solutions, the very language, how it's spoken by the varied speakers, and how it's received by the varied audiences, requires more than simple interest in collaboration. More than simple translation, even. Rather, *how* a sociologist considers race, *how* a neurologist approaches a stroke patient, *how* a rhetorician speaks to a vascular surgeon, *how* a cardiologist hears a bebop pianist can be the location of our well-intended discourse, if impotent to date.

What could we, this ragtag band of medical school deans and deputy provosts, cardiologists, professors of English, surgeons, sociologists, pediatricians, psychologists, and rhetoricians do next? What can we do that is more than bloviation and closer to concrete betterment?

Medicine, to my surprise after I'd finished clinical training, is located in political and economic contexts. But medicine can also be located in humanity, as I initially suspected, which, by all appearances and payment policies, is subordinate. An audience that is either unaware of, or indifferent to, health disparities based on race, but might otherwise find such discourse interesting, even inviting, if the very content of health disparities based on race in American medicine emerged as the crux, and not our own disciplinary jargon and ways of thinking, could help. As Shakespeare's *Hamlet* teaches us: the play's the thing.

Somehow, despite my time in Baltimore, once, I remain convinced that interdisciplinarity is required if we are to cut into these overt and tangible health disparities that began with the beginning of America and persist right through today. And tomorrow. Certainly, these disparities in health outcomes are commensurate with disparities in education, income, law enforcement, housing, etc. Then, it's no wonder that physicians, alone, are not qualified to eliminate these disparities. The Greek Tragedy of race in American history is what stands between the present and solutions to health disparities between the races. I am worried, however, that the necessary bricolage might finally disallow our roundtable.

9

Think

There's courage in the opening of "Think," Aretha Franklin's 1968 song: *You better think! Think about what you're tryin' to do to me.* A command more than a request. A warning. An exhortation with certain penalty attached for not heeding. I'm startled at the outset of her song. Then emboldened. A feminist anthem, of sorts, I sense I ought to listen. I ought to think. Maybe I've made too much of this. I suppose I like the rhythm along with the text as I consider my own stance as an audience all around: music, literature, medicine. I work to be a better audience. I first understood that I needed to become a better audience during late adolescence when I discovered my own literary limitations. I was not functionally illiterate; but was not ready, as it were, to read in college, and to think about what I was to read.

The first book I ever read read was during the second semester of the eleventh grade: *To Kill a Mockingbird*. I recall that the Black woman took the White children with her to a Black church. Because I was already too old for this to have been the first book I'd ever read, I was far behind my classmates at Berkeley during my freshman year as an undergraduate. Instead of English 1A, I decided to take Afro-American Literature 1A with my roommate and some other classmates I met during the summer before our freshman year. Of the books we read that quarter, I mainly remember Richard Wright's *Black Boy*. I don't believe I understood our professor's lecture about fiction, nonfiction, and Wright's interaction with reality, history, narration, and protest. I found that I prefer unreliable narrators. That is to say, I don't know what was actual in *Black Boy*; neither is this important to me. *How* I was to consider literature was concretized for me much later when I read a piece of nonfiction by Gabriel García Márquez where he recounted a dream that he could not be sure was a dream, and not reality. In the end, he did not consider the two conflated, but considered the two versions as one reality—the distinction between dream and reality, if it existed, was irrelevant to García Márquez.

I mainly remember one thing about the protagonist in *Black Boy*. It's when he was interested in obtaining a library card. Since Black people were not allowed to obtain library cards in his Mississippi, he needed a White person to help him. "Which of them would now help me to get books?" Jewish, Baptist, Irish Catholic? Wright went with the Irish Catholic. "Since he, too, was an object of hatred, I felt that he might refuse me but would hardly betray me." I recognized myself in the protagonist. Not at all related to religion, but to Richard Wright's scrutiny of the varied White men available in his Mississippi reality. I am like Richard Wright's protagonist in this way. I ruminate when confronted with how to choose people who might be on my side, who would hardly betray me.

I enjoyed Afro-American Studies 1A so much that I took 1B the next semester. Then, in my sophomore year, I took a survey course of Afro-American Literature. I did not know at the time that my professor, Barbara Christian, was the mother of Black Feminist Literary Criticism. She seemed interested in me, per se, and in my eagerness to become literate. I discovered a narrative that could bespeak the solitude I felt as a Mexican in America. A Mexican who'd never been to Mexico, didn't speak Spanish, was not Catholic, and had no ancestors in Mexico whom I could find, or who could find me. William Wells Brown, Harriet Wilson, Charles Chesnutt, Jean Toomer, Zora Neale Hurston, Richard Wright, Ralph Ellison, James Baldwin, Margaret Walker, Alice Walker, Toni Morrison. A real image of a brown boy from central California who was an outsider in America emerged as I read these Afro-American fictions.

Sick and Tired

I recently flew to Chicago for a luncheon ceremony celebrating my pediatrics professor, a heroine for all of us in her path. The chain Italian restaurant was packed with my professor's former students, colleagues, friends, church people, and the like. I sat at a round table of eight or ten with a dear friend from medical school, then the Deputy Provost at the University of Chicago. He waved me over to join him and his family where a few seats remained. Another Black man, whom I didn't know, also sat with them. He and I chatted about the medical event at hand, the restaurant, and any number of things I cannot now remember. I started speaking my normal bombastic discourse with this unknown Black man while our mutual friend held a child or two and listened from across the table. Evidently, I'd casually referenced Jean Toomer, Ralph Ellison, Zora Neale Hurston, Alice Walker, and so forth, during our prologue chat as we awaited the luncheon program. This Black man sitting next to me listened, probed, prompted, and questioned me as I rallied. After one of my hyperboles, he said, "Let me ask you a question: Why do you study African American Literature?" Like a jazz saxophonist high on a riff, I impulsively said, "Oh, that's easy. For two reasons." I will admit, here, that I only had one reason in mind when I responded, but thought I could conjure a second as I explained the first. If I were unable to conjure a second, I planned to talk so much about the first that he'd forget I promised more. I started: "I read Afro-American Literature—you see, it was called Afro-American when I was in college. That tells you how old I am—because, on its own, this is a worthy area of academic study. Like Chinese History or Russian Literature. No one asks Condoleezza Rice why she studied Russia because Russia is a worthy area of academic study on its own. Afro-American Literature, too, is worthy, without defense, explanation, or apology. Maybe people do ask Rice why she studied Russia. They shouldn't. Or Ruth Simmons studying French Literature." Spirited, I sat up straight. At the edge of my seat. Arms brandishing about. I'd thought of the second reason around the time I mentioned Chinese History. "And secondly, I'm a Mexican in America. But I didn't come from Mexico. My people came to America from central California. But I'm not wanted here. Then, if I'm to understand what it means to be an unwanted minority in my own country, I've got to contend with Richard Wright. I know Black people are from Africa, but they're really from Mississippi. Bigger Thomas in Chicago reminds me of myself. I then need to extrapolate what it means for Black people who are unwanted here to my own Mexicanness in America. So, if I want to know what it means to be a minority in America where I'm not wanted, but have no home country beyond Stockton, then I've got to contend with

Bigger Thomas." The Black man, a renouned surgeon, exploded, "I think of race every day and never would have come up with that one!"

The Deputy Provost sat across the table and smiled quietly as the luncheon speeches were about to begin.

The luncheon exchange occurred two years before Foghorn Leghorn (a name that my friend, Richard Rodriguez, used to help us understand the last presidential campaign) resurrected Mexican Exclusion. The election results hit the mark of this barely dormant reality capable of being promptly resurrected.

I listen to Cornel West every chance I get. I admit I don't always understand everything he says. I don't blame him. Rather, I try to become a better audience so that I might understand more the next time. Either way, I find him entirely entertaining. I laugh and I think—an important combination for me. I'd seen him on TV doing interviews, on C-SPAN panels, lecturing. My friend, a professor of English the University of the Pacific, told me that Cornel West would be speaking there, in Stockton, one evening and invited me to join her in the audience. I showed up early, without any special privilege, and stood in line among the students and professors—none of whom had any special privilege—and rushed in to get a good seat once the doors opened. Cornel West walked to the stage and began by greeting his mother, who didn't live far from Stockton, and other family members who sat in the front row. This greeting lasted much longer than I might have guessed. Indeed, the audience noticed the duration and murmured. Cornel West looked up and said, "This is family," and continued his greetings. He then walked over to the lectern and delivered a fiery sermon, which I could barely follow, but enjoyed, entirely. "The Walmartinization of America," was the funniest and smartest line I remember.

Cornel West is from Sacramento, California, the big city of my childhood, about forty miles north. He was delighted to be "home," in Stockton, not far from Sacramento, for the lecture at UOP. I saw my childhood pediatrician in the crowd, and sat with him. He and his wife knew West's parents from their undergraduate days at Fisk University in Nashville. My pediatrician jokingly remembered when Cornel West visited Fisk and kissed the ground where his parents met. "If it wasn't for this spot, I wouldn't be here."

After the lecture, which lasted almost two hours, inclusive of the salutations, some of us walked to the President's House where Cornel West was to sign some books. I sat on the couch with my pediatrician, his wife, and Cornel West's mother, who delighted us with stories about when he was a child. She noted that he was staying with her in Sacramento, and that he would be reading for several more hours after the lecture and the drive back home from Stockton. My pediatrician's wife took me through the crowd to meet Cornel West. We shook hands. I mentioned how much I enjoyed his work, and that I was working on a book about jazz and medicine. He suggested a book for me to read. I impressed him with the introduction of another that I'd read on the topic. Cornel West drifted back in to the crowd as he pointed at me, preacherly, in solidarity.

My wife attends a nearby Black church. I intermittently attend because I enjoy the singing, appreciate the lessons, and am inspired by the epideictic speech. In concert with a local university, the church brought in Cornel West on a Saturday. We sat in the middle pews among the local university students, some members of the congregation, and the church leaders. Cornel West thundered down upon us, both sermon and sociology—precisely what I'd hoped to receive. While it's difficult to remember everything he said, and impossible to capture it here, or anywhere, I recall a poignant and cautionary lesson about the "Santaclausification" of Martin Luther King, Jr.

I watched Cornel West during an interview. Maybe it was with the New York Times' Frank Rich on C-SPAN. Maybe someone else. I don't remember the details of this discussion, but was moved by a passage where he described an annual meeting he convenes with a few friends. I don't recall the names beyond Bill Bradley. As I understood the passage, this is a meeting of a few people from a variety of fields and backgrounds who gather each year to discuss the various topics or new ideas that aren't necessarily parts of their workaday jobs. This annual meeting is sort of a convention, but for themselves, not a commercial organization or a university event. This small band meets to discuss whatever it is they are respectively working through at the time such that they listen to each presentation, ask each other questions, offer alternatives, insight, and distinct ways of thinking about the topic at hand.

I thought I might convene my own group of thinkers. Some close friends loved the idea and agreed to participate. Like Richard Wright before us, we thought about who might be best-suited for this think tank that is not ratified, not sanctioned, not funded, and does not exist, save in the church air with Cornel West's words filling up the pews. We included some, excluded others, thought about yet others, added one more, removed another one, and, at this moment, are still in the throes of trying to gauge who might best constitute this elixir of thinkers.

That is, how can we choose?

As I called one, then another, they raised the perfunctory obligatory questions: What's the purpose? What would I say? Am I qualified to participate? What's the end goal? What will be the progression toward the next meeting? Are we looking to create a product? A book? A documentary? Should we seek funding? What are you doing?

The question that penetrated through this barrage was almost a mandate that a binary approach serve as the very foundation of our would-be think tank. If we do this, what will be our result? If we do that, what will be our result?

But thinking about race in America, for example, cannot be a binary equation with quantifiable, measurable, reproducible results on a spreadsheet that can be easily converted to a bar graph or a pie chart with some pivots and a right-click. Two hundred and fifty years of slavery followed by a civil war and ten years of Reconstruction did not do the trick when we consider Black people in Chicago who got there because they were run out of Mississippi during Jim Crow. A chapter in a book, beyond the meatpacking book, *The Jungle*, let's say, as it relates to modern meat inspection and the Food and Drug Administration, or possibly *Uncle Tom's Cabin* as a supplement to abolitionists prior to the U.S. Civil War, cannot be our ambition.

Think

I imagine our initial meeting in Las Vegas or Los Angeles where we can hear each other, offer criticism and insight, offer synergy and dissonance, tell of our intellectual interests and pursuits, and engage in some intelligent discourse on any number of related and unrelated topics.

We can figure out what we would do next. What would be our expected outcome of this first meeting? What would we expect of this group over the years? Documentary? Book? Just some good thoughts exchanged between smart, funny people? This would be extremely valuable if this is what we get. But what else might we try to generate? This first meeting could be a time when we decide what this group will become. We could respond to our perfunctory obligatory questions, then dismiss them.

Honestly interdisciplinary discussion. People from humanities, social science, medicine, and science can broaden our thinking. Strengthen our thinking.

Who will talk first? Who will talk next? How will we keep from getting derailed? Is it possible to get derailed in this sort of gathering? I'm interested in the role of the audience. How might I become a better audience? I might also talk about music and literature as they could (but don't) intersect with regular living and work discourse. A cardiologist might be interested in how we communicate with great superficiality in our culture as compared with intended substance. A rhetorician will consider a pipeline of Black leadership. An academic dean might consider "diversity" when looking at prestigious American boarding schools, elite small and large colleges, or even, perhaps, other areas in society where *actual* diversity is necessary for our evolution. A biomechanical engineer might apply his scientific thought process and approach to design to overtly social problems like race in America and health disparities. This one promises to be the most inventive. Maybe leadership. In any case, we will all contribute in superadditive ways—both as speakers and as the audience.

We are not yet prepared for the organic think tank, but have readied ourselves through the decades with our respective educations, careers, and our interactions with the eternal present. Like jazz soloists convening backstage after the show. This precipice will inspire our own thoughts.

Las Vegas is close. Flights are cheap. Nice hotels are cheap. Meals are cheap. We would need a room to meet. Maybe something at one of the hotels. Maybe someone will get a suite, and we could use the living room? Maybe June? Maybe winter. Not Super Bowl Weekend. We could fly to Las Vegas, let's say, on Friday, get dinner, and be ready to meet Saturday morning. Dinner Saturday night, then the rest on Sunday morning. End at Noon, or 2 p.m., or so, on Sunday, and then fly back home. We'd need to check our disciplines at the door.

10

Jesus of Exeter

We lived in a government duplex, beige with brown trim, on the south side of Stockton until the summer before the sixth grade when we moved to a small house on the other side of the new freeway, Interstate 5, from where I would walk to my new school the next academic year. Because busing from one side of town to the other in order to mix the races of elementary school children had not yet started, and because we were not naturally integrated with White children, we were Mexican, Filipino, Black, Japanese, and Chinese, for the most part, on the south side of town, alone. There was one White kid, Billy Miles, at the new school. A Filipino kid, a Black kid, and Billy Miles comprised a trio that welcomed me, an unknown Mexican, into their band.

What I remember most about Billy Miles now, forty-one years later, happened on a Monday. He had stumbled into his grandfather's Richard Pryor records and memorized, among others, a Mudbone sketch. "She had a monkey's foot around her neck, and a three-legged monkey. And that monkey didn't give her *no* trouble." I ached with laughter when I was twelve years old as Billy Miles recited the elongated Richard Pryor chronicle with precise linguistic stresses: "She squatted and pissed. That's right! She pissed for fifteen minutes. Old, strong, ammonia piss, too."

Busing to mix the races of American children started in Stockton the next year, twenty-two years after the 1954 *Brown v. Board* Supreme Court desegregation decision, when I was to start the seventh grade. We didn't get bused to White schools; we stayed on the south side while White kids were bused to us. I walked to Marshall Middle School, back into the housing projects from which I had recently emerged, and watched the buses on that first day of school as they arrived with White kids from the north side. There were no incidents like the ones I'd later learn about when busing in Boston started, for example, which would have been an inverse of Black, Filipino, Mexican, Chinese, and Japanese parents shouting obscene epithets at White children descending upon south Stockton. Nothing happened. We went to class, became friends throughout middle school, and later found that the White kids whose parents had enough money, and were concerned about mixing the races of children, had either entered their children into private schools or moved to different neighborhoods that did not require busing to our school, and did not send their teenagers to our south side high school.

Aside from the would-be integration that busing offered, the Physical Education classes had integrated the genders by then. Of course, the locker rooms were segregated by gender, but the actual gym class was a mix of boys and girls. Black girls, Chinese girls, Filipino boys, Mexican boys, Japanese girls, Mexican girls, Black boys, and so forth. As numeric minority children in America who'd grown up oblivious to our minority status because we were all we knew, grown-up racial distinctions did not concern us. The Chinese girl who was to become our valedictorian enjoyed sports more than the rest of us boys. Indeed, during the basketball section of gym class, she was a top draft pick when choosing teams. I recall her posting up a tall, Black boy down low. I sent her an entry pass. She faked, pivoted, turned, and threw a sky hook along the lines of Kareem Abdul-Jabbar over the tall Black boy's outstretched arm. I cannot recall whether she expressed trash talking, which makes this story better, or whether this only exists in my mind. In the end, whether this trash talking actually happened is unrelated to my reality: it's forever embedded in my mind. "In your face!"

I'm old enough to have gone to college when we were only allowed to apply to one University of California campus. I'd planned to apply to UCLA because it was far from Stockton and I'd seen their famous basketball team on TV. That was my entire analysis of any college prospects. My English teacher encouraged me to switch my application from UCLA to UC Berkeley, his alma mater, and explained Berkeley's muscle to me. I followed his advice because it was the only advice I received about college. I was accepted at Berkeley. I was also invited to join a summer program set up for "underrepresented minority" students to help us enter what Berkeley understood to be a foreign land—even if we had not yet understood this. Summer Bridge. A nostalgic time where I would spend my classroom days with students who, for the last time, reminded me of my neighborhood. Smart Mexican and Black pre-freshman walked through Sather Gate, up and down Telegraph Avenue, tie-dyed T-shirts of yore, days of protesting one thing or another. Leopald's Records. Blondie's Pizza. Top Dog!

The first day of fall quarter was the very first time in my life that I felt like a minority. I understood the numeric realities of Mexicans in California, but had not yet understood that these numerators and denominators—fractions of people—could evoke in me such an alien emotional sense. A stranger in the village, like James Baldwin in Switzerland. I looked at the swell of White people, my Berkeley classmates, on that first day, paralyzed. Frantically, I looked around for my Summer Bridge classmates. I saw one in the distance, also looking around. Then another. Then more. We gathered on Telegraph Avenue and started to enjoy the morning. Some of us didn't make it to through to graduation from Berkeley. Some went on to graduate or professional school and lived lives commensurate with what anyone might think Berkeley graduates might live, independent of race.

I spent the summer before medical school in a program analogous to Summer Bridge where racial minority students met each other, became familiar with the medical school campus, and began a momentum that would sustain us through the medical school fray. I joined both the Latino and the Black medical school clubs because I was friends with both groups from our summer session, and because I understood from my undergraduate sociology and Ethnic Studies classes, and from my childhood in south Stockton, that this is smart. I'm not certain, but I recall that our Dean of Student Affairs was the only Black dean in the country, save the Black medical schools. In any case, during this summer session before medical school was to start, he required that we sit in the front rows of the lecture hall. "You can see better, you won't be distracted, and you look like you belong," he reasoned with us.

Though none of us planned to sit in the front rows once fall started, we naturally entered class on the first day and returned to "our" summer seats in the front of the lecture hall. During one of the racist episodes later in the year, the dean met with the class to discuss the tension. One of the White students said something about "*their* seats in front." Without getting into the trite details of that particular racist episode, or any of the others, I recognized that the White student, more than us, considered those to be *our* seats. I later invited her to join us in the front, where we could see, where we would not be distracted, where we looked like we belonged.

My wife and I chose to move our children to a White and Asian city because the public schools were touted as some of the best in the state. When our two eldest children were in elementary school, there were a total of four Black and four Mexican children in the entire school from K – 6th grades. I quipped to a friend, "There are four Mexican kids, and two of them are ours. There are four Black kids, and two of them are ours. Our kids comprise 50% of *both* the Mexican and Black kids in the entire school!" Maybe this wasn't a quip.

Dissatisfied with the social and academic possibilities (perhaps fodder for another book), we later moved these two children to private schools. In our daughter's freshman class were five Black students: a Nigerian girl, a Black boy from Los Angeles, and three others, including our daughter, who might have to narrate their Blackness with a simple pedigree from genetics textbook chapter about round and wrinkled peas, if they were even interested in explaining to anyone that they are Black.

We looked at some of the esteemed boarding schools on the east coast when our son later looked to enter high school. Some of the schools' students provided oratory about their experiences far away from home, about the rigors of the education at prestigious boarding schools, and answered questions from parents in the audience who were worried about sending their children away for high school. We arrived a little early to one of the receptions, but were unable to find the meeting room, which was on the top floor of a west Los Angeles hotel. One of the desk clerks discovered that the reception was on the top floor and pointed me and my wife to the express elevator located around the corner from the bank of main elevators. This allowed us to rise directly to the top floor, unfettered by stops along the way up.

During the recruiting presentation, an especially insightful and eloquent Mexican senior student who'd grown up in a dangerous part of central Los Angeles spoke of the riches of his education in the hotel's top floor reception. Perfectly poised, he allowed the boarding school administrator and the sophomore students to respond, but was able to read the audience and chip in when he understood the exchange to be deficient. Impressive. By the end of the evening, after all of the questions and concerns had been addressed, we left the room. Privileged to know about the express elevator, my wife and I rounded the corner away from the main bank of elevators where we found the Mexican student waiting to take the express elevator down to the bottom. He looked up and greeted us. I told him how impressed we were with his eloquence and substance. Humble, he smiled. He asked if we had any further questions he could answer.

Playfully, I asked, "How do you get a Mexican from the bad part of LA to Exeter?"

He confessed to us in a tone that differed from his poise onstage, solemn, with notes of melancholy: "Sometimes I feel alone."

I called my friend, a Black surgeon, whose son went to a different east coast boarding school, and asked how his son fared. I asked whether we should send our California son way out east. My friend said about his son's experience, "He's never been around Black kids who've never been around Black kids."

We decided that our son should stay home, in California, as a fourteen-year-old boy. We would supplement his education: Ralph Ellison, James Baldwin, Toni Morrison, August Wilson, Juan Rulfo, Gabriel García Márquez, Richard Rodriguez, and the others.

Our third child remains in public school. Her class is filled with Korean, Chinese, and Indian children. Indians, somehow, became Asians over the course of my life. Our daughter looks Indian. Either from Calcutta or Mesoamerica, or from prehistoric and modern California.

I briefly worked in Connecticut a few years ago when we first considered moving our family to the east coast. I drove to Bridgeport for a morning meeting. I had an afternoon meeting scheduled, and didn't want to drive back to the remote hotel between meetings. The executive assistant walked me to the front of the building at the end of the morning meeting and pointed me to the garage where I'd parked. I asked her where I might go for lunch so that I could sit and pass the time before my afternoon meeting. She asked what kind of food I liked. "Anything" I said. She pointed to a restaurant on the corner of the next block. "We go there most of the time. It's good." I asked what kind of food the restaurant served. "Spanish," she said. Considering this foreign restaurant, I wondered about any other options that might be available to me. I asked if there were any other places she could recommend. She turned and pointed in the opposite direction and said that there was another good restaurant around that corner. I asked what kind of food they served. Again, she said, "Spanish." I was honestly confused, and abruptly asked a clarifying question: "You mean from Spain?" In an attempt to end this line of questioning forever, she asked, "What are you?" "Mexican." "You'll like it. Rice and beans." I thanked the executive assistant and waited until she went back into the building. I walked to my car and drove to McDonald's where I ate a familiar combo meal and waited for my afternoon meeting.

Sometimes I feel alone. Misplaced Mexicans or abandoned Nigerian graduate students or Black boarding school children are singular, modern examples of our failure to achieve the reified promise of America. We are not always seen as full-bodied human beings, despite our progress. Neither am I interested in being seen by someone else. This would solve nothing. I am an outsider. Alterity has become a comfortable location for me. If I'm interchangeable with a Coeur d'Alene Indian, a Filipino girl, a Black man from Oakland, and a Ghanaian from London, an Asian (Korean? Cantonese? Taiwanese?), a Dominican, and a peroxide blonde Hispanic, then who will accept that Russian poet Joseph Brodsky is my inspiration, that I read Nikolai Gogol, that I believe Dostoyevsky wrote for me?

Diversity, a treacherous word, for all its good intentions, is understood to be a key part of the small bag of tricks toward solutions to health disparities. The profound superficiality, with its cowardly attempts at diversity, ensure that colorful people comply with those who allowed them inside. That is, we can be different colors provided we concede a natural subordination, lest we be disallowed. I mean to say that if the sensibility of a solitary Black medical student in a White medical school in the 1940s is replicated in the 1960s, the 1980s, last year, and next year, then there is no hope that diversity, itself, can be understood as a solution to health outcomes disparities based on race.

The modern minority feels alone up there on the top floor of a west side hotel.

A public health pediatrician notes that the Black infant mortality rate is more than twice the rate of the White infant mortality rate, and has not changed from the time she entered medicine until her recent retirement. Then, more diversity is not the answer. Of course, I'm in favor of diversity; but a New Zealander or a Dubliner or a Scot or a Londoner with her origins in Ghana would all provide diversity, per se, but would be anemic when considering the inevitable differences in human decay when we look at Mexicans working the vegetable fields or in the executive board rooms, or when looking at Black babies simply being born, for example.

I am a dislocated Mexican from Stockton. Geographically, socially, culturally isolated. It's easier, more sterile, to capture me in a spreadsheet, along with the Cockney African and the Moroccan in the outskirts of Paris, than to examine the underbelly of educating poor minority children. Alas, I've come to understand that there never was an intention to land upon a real solution for honest desegregation—let alone integration, acceptance, and humanity. I gained an insight to health disparities based on race when I watched Gunter Grass, the Nobel Prize winner in literature, respond to a question about why Germany *actually* changed after WWII. Grass let the interviewer finish his languid question and then said, "The defeat of Germany was complete."

What went wrong in America after the promise of freedom after the Civil War, after the 1960s, after the childhood summers that promised an elusive humanity? Where did the humanity go that would be horrified by the persistently high Black infant mortality rate? Horrified enough to act? Should Black babies die at a high rate without our outrage? Without our action, since outrage is not enough? There are plenty of stories about how America never found its way when it comes to race. We are inconsolable because in this Greek Tragedy America deliberately walked off of a virtuous path, highlighted in lofty prose, and never attained our nationhood because this was never her ambition—not at the outset, not after the Civil War, not after the 1960s.

That is, the defeat of mistreating people of different races in America was not complete. Not the way Gunter Grass meant about Germany.

Bryan Stevenson, Executive Director of the Equal Justice Initiative in Montgomery, Alabama, in a reference to Nelson Mandela and the post-apartheid era of Truth and Reconciliation, notes that America has not ever dealt with the *truth* part, and, therefore, *cannot* get to the reconciliation part. A *New York Times* article notes fewer underrepresented minority students in elite colleges now when compared to the mid-1980s, and can be understood as an argument in favor of diversity in colleges and medical schools if real solutions are America's intent. The last few decades have proven that this approach is wrong: the so-called "underrepresented minority" medical and pre-medical students as "the" answer to the perennial disparities in Black infant mortality rate. My friends in medicine and I, slated to fill this role, carry the weight of national tensions that originate in our origins a few centuries ago. We struggle to breathe deeply in our solitude.

Part Three

The Audience and New Ideas

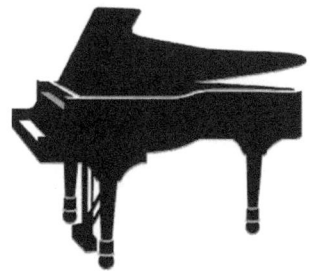

11

Two Instants

Chinatown, with its Tang Dynasty facades and big storefront windows that allow tourists to see inside, and owners to see outside, rests across the street from San Francisco's modern financial district skyscrapers. An old man sits on a corner playing an erhu—a thousand-year-old two-string fiddle with a bow. Tourists stop to listen. Some throw coins into his jar. Teenagers smoke against the wall. I walk past the dim sum place where President Obama once ate. "Go to the other one. It's quieter. Just as good. You can have a conversation. But you won't see President Obama."

I began my new job as a physician executive in Chinatown with a new-employee physical exam at a local clinic. The Chinese medical assistant measured my height, weight, pulse, and blood pressure. She then escorted me to an examination room where I was to wait for the Chinese physician. In English, she asked if I would like some hot water. I said, "For what?" The demure Chinese medical assistant bowed slightly and said, "In our culture, it is customary to offer hot water." Brash, I asked, "You mean like for some tea?" Agreeably, "Well, yes, you can add tea. Or you can drink the hot water without tea." More excitedly than I should have, I said, "Hot water by itself! No. I don't want any hot water." The assistant smiled and left me alone to wait. I thought about the hot water exchange and recognized that I, a Mexican originally from central California, didn't understand what just *happened*.

Chinatown, not far from the Golden Gate Bridge, the San Francisco Giants' new baseball stadium, Fisherman's Wharf, the new technology satellite Mecca, Union Square, Moscone Center—not far from anything in San Francisco—exists against the backdrop of the past century and a half. Patients simply walk into the health insurance Member Services office with questions about anything at all. Many elderly don't understand how to even access healthcare outside of Chinatown. Dialing a number and following a phone tree is impossible. If the call is in English, they will simply hang up. Some walk in with their mail asking for help sorting it. This is a critical step in providing healthcare. An employee segregates the mail into junk, electric, gas, phone bills, and other pieces, including mail from his doctor. Here is where particular, tangible help is delivered by the staff in Cantonese: critical lab results, cancer screening tests to be scheduled, primary care appointments, a heating bill. The patient holds out an unopened envelope and asks in Cantonese, "What is it?" The staff cannot say, "We are only your health insurance plan." They are obligated to help because the envelope's contents could be important. The patient recognizes a dollar sign and asks, "How much do I owe you? I couldn't sleep last night. Couldn't eat. I hope I don't owe you *this* much."

This is not a simplistic question of language. Not a sterile translation of English, a Germanic language written in a Latin alphabet, into Chinese characters. This is not even a verbal exchange in Cantonese that describes what's written, in either language. It's more *pragmatics*, a branch of linguistics, than medicine. An employee from Hong Kong whose primary language is Cantonese, though she is also fluent in Mandarin and English, explained to me that if she is speaking in Mandarin with someone from northern China who asks her a question, she would understand his question completely, would answer accurately, and would be completely understood by the northern Chinese man. "I got an A in Mandarin! But I would have no idea *why* he is asking that question." The Chinatown patient's health is located inside of his social and cultural reality, and is then translated into health. Or else, it is not. "He needs to know what is *happening*. This may be the difference in human life." The patient needs a cancer screening, the electricity bill is overdue, the dollar sign is only an explanation of benefits such that he does *not* owe any money. This last part is repeated at least three times in Cantonese. The member gathers his mail and prepares to leave. "I can sleep tonight."

Chinatown has been peppered with disruptive events that required Chinese people to turn inward, to help themselves, in order to survive. Opium Wars, civil war, hunger, and indestructable poverty contributed to southern China emigration to San Francisco where cheap labor was prized in the 1850s, like it is today. The continuum of standard violence, the Chinese Exclusion Act of 1882, the 1906 earthquake, and the chronology of affronts through today prompted Chinese people in San Francisco to remain resolute, if they were to live. Not as hyperbolic locution, but as actual, physical survival.

In addition to the everlasting Chinese people, some over one hundred years old, who landed in San Francisco to work—restaurants, railroads, laundry, agriculture—new poor Chinese immigrants, like their predecessors, for nearly the same reasons, now arrive in San Francisco. Then, the same self-help impetus exists.

Add to this century and half continuum the most recent seismic event to intersect with healthcare in Chinatown: The Affordable Care Act. This creates a new cadence in the healthcare arc in Chinatown by including Whites, Mexicans, Central Americans, and more who are now able to purchase newly available health insurance. New patients speak English, Spanish, Vietnamese, Mandarin, Cambodian, Russian, and so forth. What's at stake in the urgent present are two competing realities: maintaining the *necessary history* of healthcare in Chinatown such that continued high-quality, culturally congruent healthcare can be delivered to existing Chinese people, and, at once, adjusting to the new and varied people who are urgently upon the healthcare capacity. A line from William Faulkner's *Light in August* offers a sense of the inescapable non sequitur in Chinatown today: "Already he can feel the two instants about to touch: the one which is the sum of his life, which renews itself between each dark and dusk, and the suspended instant out of which the *soon* will presently begin."

A Spanish-speaking Nicaraguense is diagnosed with diabetes. An English-speaking Mexican is screened for cancer. A White man takes his son for vaccines. A nurse tells me about an eighty-four-year-old Chinese woman from Vietnam who came to visit her aunt and never left San Francisco. All of the Chinese woman's family, refugees in Vietnam after the Japanese invasion of China during WWII, had already died. No husband, no children. The

San Francisco aunt died, leaving the Chinese woman from Vietnam with no familial connection anywhere on earth. Her aunt had arranged for some people to give the Chinese woman $500 each month. The woman's rent is $450 each month. She gets one meal each day from a benevolent association in Chinatown. She eats half of the meal at noon, and saves the other half for dinner. The organization ordinarily expects a $2 donation for meals, but waived the price for this woman. Proud, the woman negotiated her way up from nothing to fifty cents per day because she thought she should pay something to live. The old woman doesn't know her relationship to the philanthropic people who come to her house to give the $500 each month. "Are they the aunt's children? That would make them the old woman's cousins." "The woman is forgetful, and doesn't know who these people are, but doesn't want to ask." I worry that the $500 will stop someday. The nurse calls various social agencies, food banks, and local groups who might be able to help. The people who give the woman money each month, and the nurses and social workers of Chinatown's healthcare collective call around daily on her behalf—an internal collective developed over the last 150 years *especially for her*—are all the Chinese woman has left on earth.

I know how this story will end. Old, sick, poorly nourished, she will soon die alone, with no earthly family.

Maybe some cousins; maybe not. Then, the remainder of her life is what's at stake for *us* now.

Why would an existing organization set out to transform itself into a guise that could provide healthcare to other people? Alterity, itself, is deceptive these days. "The other" is utterly rejected in our country's history. Still, we speak the *idea* of difference as if it's desired. Business schools tout the "minority" voice as curative against corporate groupthink; the Supreme Court (old and new cases) wrestle with "race" from antiquity, and from today, as We the People wonder to whom we are referring, if not us all.

Diversity is all the new rage.

But diversity so that dissenting opinions in businesses might generate greater profits, and the one Black kid at a private school who is on the cover of the brochure, misses the substance when considering outcomes of flesh, heartbeats, leg amputations from complications of untreated diabetes. The Affordable Care Act requires that we pay attention to health inequalities. Some state regulators require answers about health outcomes disparities from health insurance companies when bidding for business. Employers who pay for their employees' healthcare understand that sicker people cost more money. Black and brown people are sicker such that improving their health outcomes ought to be financially attractive to the corporate class.

Sick and Tired

Whether to address health inequalities on pecuniary, ethical, or humanitarian grounds is not in question. Rather, *how* to achieve such concrete betterment, after the last few centuries, remains up in the air.

A simple call to Member Services by someone whose primary language is Spanish is answered by someone whose primary language is Cantonese. Both speak English—each with her respective accent—but do not really understand each other. This intersection is not simply different languages, and it's more than accents and broken English. This is not a question of language translation, but of two versions of reality.

Can healthcare that is overtly and tangibly rooted in the historic reality of Chinese people of yore be spread, "scaled," to places outside of Chinatown? Can it successfully expand to include new membership brought by new laws? If its own history is the crux of the care provided to Chinese people in San Francisco, which has extended to surrounding areas over the last few decades, and *now* includes non-Chinese, non-Cantonese-speaking people as its "community," then the present must conflate with the past toward this end.

We are to *do* something in that space between Faulkner's two instants, the urgent present, that results in the old call for concrete betterment now—especially now—that we are able to live, and know what is happening, and recognize each other.

Two Instants

* * *

When he was a medical student at UCLA, my friend, along with his fellow Muslim classmates, started a clinic not far from Florence and Normandy in South Central Los Angeles. This section of LA connotes Black people who relocated from Texas and the Deep South, the Watts Riots of 1965, and the Rodney King Riots of 1992. It is now interchangeable, in fact, with Mexicans and Central Americans. Perhaps as part of new clandestine gentrification, I was struck when I saw a White couple at Woody's BBQ, not far from Florence and Normandy. I don't know if they were struck to see me.

* * *

We enrolled our youngest daughter in ballet. We chose The Debbie Allen Dance Academy (DADA), established on Crenshaw Boulevard in Los Angeles by the famous dancer-actress-choreographer-producer-director, Debbie Allen, and her husband, former Los Angeles Laker, Norm Nixon. Created on Crenshaw to fill a void for the children there, and anywhere, who might learn the language of dance as hope. We enrolled our youngest daughter in four classes: Ballet, Tap, Hip Hop, and African. I drove her to class on that first Saturday and noticed a movie billboard sign, as large as life, right in front of DADA:

Straight Outta Compton in black and white. We live in a Taiwanese-Korean-Indian-White area of southern California. DADA is a laminar reality for our privileged daughter. This is also true for her classmates on Crenshaw. An interior reality required to weather the exterior one. I like the name DADA, like Dada, the artistic form challenging conformity in favor of freedom.

* * *

I worry that I'm writing about a foreign land. One I would not recognize. One where I might not readily understand the culture. But this new land is what I've come to fancy, isn't it? The first time my wife and I went skiing was uneventful, to my surprise. I did not fall down a slippery slope. I did not run into a tree. We drove to a Lake Tahoe resort unprepared, entirely. I believe I wore blue jeans. We stood in the lobby of the rental office trying to decide whether to rent skis and purchase bunny slope lessons. Or should we leave and rent tire innertubes and sled down a gentle hill instead? We stood back, not at the ready, not next in line, but amorphous in the lobby looking at the menu of rental possibilities. No one addressed us. No one noticed us. We had nothing about which to complain. After some time, I felt out of place. Though I've never been to a frat house beyond watching *Animal House* again and again, I imagined this is how I'd feel there: out of place. This *place* is a question for me. Not longitude and latitude. Then what? Where I belong; and where I might have the freedom to go. This place was not built for me. Did not have me in mind. I tense when someone asks about my writing, "Who's your intended audience?" I drift off and wonder if Dostoyevsky might have answered, "A Mexican medical student in the future I cannot know." I doubt this. We rented skis, declined the lessons, and swished down the slight incline slowly. My jeans were soaked, in the end.

* * *

I watched a WWII movie. I can't remember which one it was. Maybe *Saving Private Ryan*. Maybe *The Pianist*. Maybe *Schindler's List*. In any case, there was a perennial scene where the Nazis ran through the streets shooting fleeing people. The ones already shot lay dead in the streets as the Nazi soldiers ran past them, chasing the ones they had not yet shot. Some on the ground were dead, to be sure. Perhaps some lay still, playing dead, hoping to elude death. Still others crawled a few feet forward, as the Nazis ran passed them and did not shoot them again, but pressed forward chasing the others still running. Death was imminent within a few feet for the ones crawling forward, both knew. I was drawn to the ones on the ground, death certain within a few feet, still crawling forward, toward human existence.

* * *

I watch a CBS *60 Minutes* segment, "The Sea Gypsies," about the Moken people, a tribe that has lived for hundreds of years on boats in the Andaman Sea about the archipelago off the coast of Myanmar. They are, of all the peoples of the world, among the least touched by modern civilization. This area has been closed to foreigners for fifty years. It is now open. The Moken are threatened with this step toward monotony of cultures. Just before the tsunami on December 26, 2004, they notice that the sea recedes away from land far into the distance. An old man tells of a campfire legend that tells of the waves: "Waters flood the earth, destroy it, make it clean again." Elephants flee for higher ground. Dolphins flee for deeper seas. The Moken survive the tsunami because they know it is coming. Long before the tsunami hits, like the elephants, they head for higher ground. They don't understand why everyone doesn't head for higher ground, as the legend recommends. The reporter asks the Moken language translator, "How old is this gentleman." The reporter answers, "He doesn't know. Time is not the same concept as we have. You can't say, for instance, 'when,' in Moken language. 'When' does not exist. 'Take' exists. And 'give.'"

12
I Can Bleed for Myself

My teenage daughter and I recently saw August Wilson's *Gem of the Ocean* at a regional theater near our home in southern California. This play, set in 1904, is the first in "The Pittsburg Cycle" of ten plays about Black people in America, one set in each decade of the twentieth century. Though it was the penultimate play August Wilson wrote, *Gem of the Ocean* initiates the twentieth century cycle. The drama considers the lives of Black people in the decades just after slavery as the drama between older characters, who had been slaves, and younger characters, who had not been slaves, emerges. My wife and I had seen *Gem of the Ocean* about ten years earlier, during its first run in Los Angeles, before it went to Broadway, starring Phylicia Rashad as the protagonist, Aunt Esther, who is 285 years old—born around the same time slavery in America was born. Our daughter, a high school senior, and I discussed this play, in particular, among the other plays she's either seen or read.

Because she is a serious student of literature, creative writing, and social justice, I did not intend for this to be an elementary discussion.

She said, "I liked the connection between jazz, current events (in the 1920s), and history in *Ma Rainey's Black Bottom*. I liked *The Piano Lesson* because the conflict between preserving one's history while working toward a better future interests me."

I asked her what she thought of *Gem of the Ocean*. She said she liked the play, but thought the first section was too sentimental. I thought of this word, "sentimental," as a serious literary criticism, and not a colloquial adolescent answer. I asked what she meant by that in a literary context. My daughter noted that the characters' dialogue and long narratives seemed to deviate from the story, itself, distracting her from the play as they talked about their feelings, not part of the drama's arc, as she saw things. I appreciated her take, and then asked her a Socratic question: "The older characters, as of 1904, were former slaves. Do you think it's asking too much of the audience to allow former slaves a chance to express their feelings and get a little TLC on Broadway? They don't have many other chances for this in the theater. Maybe a little in the First Act of an August Wilson play isn't too much to ask?"

My teenage daughter agreed with me, which isn't altogether common.

I Can Bleed for Myself

She asked which was my favorite. Though it is his most popular play, August Wilson said during an interview that he didn't like *Fences* as much as the rest of us. His favorite was *Joe Turner's Come and Gone* because of its nationalism, it's self-reliance. He especially liked his great line, spoken by the protagonist, Herald Loomis, "I don't need nobody to bleed for me! I can bleed for myself," before he takes a knife to his own chest.

I like *Fences*. I also like Wilson's final play, *Radio Golf*, which integrates some of the characters from previous plays, including *Gem of the Ocean*, another favorite of mine. Like August Wilson, I also love the self-reliance of *Joe Turner's Come and Gone*, and that great line. My favorite, however, is probably *The Piano Lesson*. I appreciate the requisite reliance on the ancestors carved into the family piano as Boy Willie fights Sutter's ghost. My favorite part is in Act 1, scene 2 when Wining Boy says, "The colored man can't fix nothing with the law." Boy Willie responds, "I don't go by what the law say. The law's liable to say anything. I go by if it's right or not. It don't matter what the law say. I take and look at it for myself."

The first Olympics I remember were the 1976 summer games in Montreal. Fourteen-year-old Nadia Comăneci, who is almost three years older than me, scored a Perfect 10 on the uneven bars. Because no one in the entire history of the Modern Olympics, which started in 1894, had ever scored a 10, there was no need for the electronic scoreboard to be equipped to show a 10. Until then. When she completed her routine on the parallel bars perfectly, the electronic scoreboard, after an unduly long delay, showed 1.00, a score that baffled me, the audience. I don't recall the details, but I'm certain that the TV broadcast announcer and other officials, too, were baffled. The announcer later explained the oversight by the scoreboard designers whose version of reality did not yet contain 10. Satisfied, I went on to enjoy the other 10's by both Comăneci and Nellie Kim, a Soviet gymnast who looked more like my Chinese friends in Stockton than the Russians I'd seen on TV. I recently watched a clip of Kim and found that her father was Korean, and Kim was not at all Chinese. Though she spoke some English during the interview, she mostly gave her answers in Russian to an English language translator.

My friends and classmates from kindergarten right on through to high school graduation were mainly Filipino, Chinese, Japanese, Mexican, and Black. It never occurred to me that any substantive differences existed between any of us. Neither did I ever think that we were simply interchangeable. Academic achievement, intelligence, speed on the track, basketball jump shots, baseball base-stealing, tennis backhands, verbal sparring, wit, rhetorical prowess, or any other aspect of childhood doesn't conjure differences based on race or ethnicity in my mind. I'd gone away to college before Vietnamese, Cambodian, and Laotian families moved to Stockton. I don't recall any Pakistani people from those days. In any case, I move freely when I visit home: my cousin's Cambodian husband and their son, my nephew, who is both White and Mexican, his White and Japanese wife, and their children, my other nephew, who is both Black and Mexican, his White wife, and their son, and so forth, including some I can't reliably describe.

That is, I easily and readily integrate with any mix of people, as far as I can tell. When I applied for a job as the medical director of a health insurance plan in San Francisco's Chinatown, for example, I spoke with the comfort I had when speaking with my elementary school classmates. By the end of the interview, I could tell things had gone well, and we were winding down the conversation about how I might fit into Chinatown, and about when I might be available to start. One of the senior executives noted that he liked the idea that I was *not* Chinese because I could exert a different influence on the medical community. I said that I am tough because I am from Stockton. He said, "Good, because this is Chinatown." I felt a little nervous, for the first time, and then left the interview more alert.

I'd already read about physician-patient congruence, cultural competence, language competence, and such, as they relate to health disparities. Of course, if a patient speaks Cantonese, and not English, speaking Cantonese when taking care of her is in order. Regrettably, this is the mainstay of discussion about health disparities. Diversity among medical students and practicing physicians is promoted as a mainstay for such congruence en route to eliminating health outcomes disparities. Or else, "cultural competence" and language translation for incongruent doctors, which solves for cultural incompetence, is another resort.

Patients prefer physicians congruent with their own culture, language, style of living. This is found at every turn in medical articles on the topic of patient-physician "congruence." I find this at every turn in ordinary life, as well. My friends and I, in our twenties, stood together at another friend's wedding reception. My uncle from across the reception hall saw us, walked over, and said, "Two Black guys and two Mexican guys standing around are either fighting or having a good time. Either way, I'm going over there!" We all laughed. Tribal enclaves that make up our "integrated" country have had to take care of each other from the interior: Chinese immigrants to San Francisco during the 1850s in their Halls of Great Peace where they went to die; Black people during Jim Crow, ordinary segregation that prohibited them from receiving healthcare in hospitals made for Whites only; current clinics and private offices in Mexican neighborhoods where Spanish is required to treat both old and new Mexicans; Cambodian patients who only see Cambodian physicians, even in emergencies; Korean people who are cared for by Korean physicians in concert with the patients' health and social needs.

Now, in the present of modern America, a required interior understanding of groups of people effectively cut off from healthcare outside of their cultural reality is, at once, an indictment of a health "system" that doesn't bother to close the chasm in health outcomes between the races, and hope because these enclaves keep struggling in our present otherness born centuries ago when our lives, like now, were dispensable.

13

Seeing Norman Lear

I delivered a sixth grade graduation speech at my elementary school after I'd become a pediatrician. A teacher thought I'd be "perfect" as a speaker for these poor children who might see that they, too, could survive poverty and live substantive professional lives someday far into their little futures. I wasn't sure how to prepare. Of course, I understood that a graduation speech should be intended for the audience of graduates, and not their parents. I've been through enough of my own graduations to know when the speakers fail. Indeed, I cannot recall a successful one. This concerned me as the next speaker up.

Though I was not preparing a talk for college or medical school graduates, I did sense a responsibility to say something that would help, that would be at least interesting in the present, and, if I were optimistic, I might even say something that would last. It's this last part that paralyzed me precisely because I was from this school, this neighborhood, these people. I worried that school, alone, without the surrounding social accoutrements required for scholarly success for these poor children who were like me in every way, would not lead them out. I don't mean to besmirch the people who've succeeded alone, in spite of their surroundings, without any help at all, unlike me. Rather, since such success from here is rare, beyond measure, I wanted to be sure I spoke to the ordinary children who were captured in the sentiment of the invitation for me to speak at all: they can make it out. However, this is not really true, by and large, when I consider the millions like them, which included me when I was at our mutual little school, separated by thirty, or so, eternal years. Then, I had another audience with whom I must contend: their parents. Alas, there were two audiences for my one speech.

Quite the conundrum.

I arrived on the late morning with some heavy things to say. While onstage, a little too late, I recognized the trap: the multiple audience. What I had prepared was more relevant to the parent audience. I was conflicted, while already talking onstage, because this was their children's graduation day. In the end, I admit, I failed as a speaker.

I recall my own sixth grade year fondly. I spent each Saturday night at my grandmother's apartment where we watched *All in the Family*. She had many other grandchildren, my cousins, but none stayed with her the way I did. What I remember most about my grandmother is that she laughed *each week* during the opening theme song, "Those were the Days," when Edith got to her screeching part: "And you knew who you *WERE* then." My grandmother laughed each Saturday night, anew, as if this were the first time she'd heard Edith's screech. Maybe not. Maybe she thought it was funny each time. Whether she'd heard it before, from one week to the next, made no difference. That's the year she died. My grandmother was old, as far as I could tell as a child, when she died. My brother and I slept in bunk beds for a few months while she lay dying in the hospital bed in our bedroom. I was young, only twelve years old, unaware of race back then. I didn't think that Edith was singing to two audiences: me and my grandmother. I didn't consider the content of *All in the Family*, its confrontation of American race the way I do now, through memory, and in the present, wrestling race to the ground. Losing, still. Then, Norman Lear addressed multiple audiences: me then, my Mexican grandmother, and the various audiences related to the Vietnam War, feminism, race, class . . . and me now.

My struggle to reach the multiple audience—students, parents, teachers—is as an example of treacherous rhetorical landscape when attempting to talk to a diverse audience, the most important part of the rhetorical triad: speaker, speech, audience. This is proving to be especially treacherous as America misses in its feeble attempts at a corrective discourse on race, in general, and in its deficient attempts to close the gap in health outcomes between races, in particular.

A few days after the last presidential election, I took my wife and children to see a lecture about race on television. Norman Lear, the creator of *All in the Family*, and Kenya Barris, the creator of *black-ish,* spoke at a fine Los Angeles middle school. We sat in the second row of the auditorium as the speakers sat a few feet in front of us, facing the audience of parents and middle school students. (I think I saw Norman Lear a few years earlier in the audience on Broadway. Maybe it was at *The Allergist's Wife*. Or else *The Beauty Queen of Leenane*. I recognized the hat. Maybe it wasn't him. He looked familiar.) The moderator at the middle school asked a question about how *All in the Family* got started. This distracted from my own expectations for the talk because Lear answered her question plainly, and spoke of the origins of the show, and how his career in television began. He eventually returned to race on TV, the topic we went to hear.

Kenya Barris responded in a way I had not yet considered, but understood instantly. He noted that his children were not as Black as he was during his own childhood; however, their White friends were Blacker than the White children of his childhood. Barris recognized that current Black and White kids were all black-ish. I looked at our own children, who are, themselves, black-ish, and laughed along with the mixed crowd. The moderator, in what seemed to be an attempt at continuing the momentum on race, then asked Norman Lear if he thought Archie Bunker could be successful today. On the next beat, Lear cooly motioned forward with his forefinger and replied, "He's gonna be president."

The varied crowd roared.

The multiple audience at the school: parents who grew up watching Norman Lear shows, and their children who are growing up watching *black-ish*. It is tricky to reach multiple audiences in the same speech. Lear, mentor to Barris, offered us a master class.

I delivered a lecture on race and medicine at a medical school a few years ago. The audience was comprised of medical students (1st, 2nd, and 4th year—the 3rd year students must have been on hospital rotations), junior faculty, senior faculty, and several medical school deans. I thought my lecture would be reasonable because by then I had learned to consider multiple echelons of understanding from each strata of a medical audience. I understood that I could say some things that would be over the heads of the early medical students, but would be rudimentary to the senior faculty. I considered a distinction in what I might say to a varied audience because of my early failures as a speaker. I understood that I could not simply water down the discourse so that the common denominators will follow because the multiple audience instantly would become uninterested. As would I. Neither could I orate thunderously about the intersection of race, history, medicine, and injustice at a noon lecture over free pizza because I was a guest, and didn't want to disturb any fledgling progress on race that might be under way. Rather, I thought I might consider where each audience member might be, and talk with them there, where they were, about health disparities based on race. Then, it would not be the chasm of a liver lecture, for example, that confused the first-year medical student, and was, at once, tiresome, to the hepatologist. Not a preachy tirade about Chronic Obstructive Pulmonary Disease to an intern and the Chief of Pulmonology. I opted, instead, to attempt something that would reach them all, and offer something substantive about race in a way that would appeal to the multiple audience.

    I worried, however, that a speech about race would be difficult since everyone is already a self-proclaimed expert on race.

I recalled some advice I received from a friend, the Chair of a small college English Department, when I asked him what he thought I might say about my best man at his funeral where I was to give the eulogy. The Chair, a medieval English scholar, advised: "Tell them something they don't know." I kept these words about my best man's death in mind as I prepared for my medical school lecture on race.

When I finished, one of the medical students I'd met as people entered the room asked a sensitive, incisive question about how doctors can spend a long time with each patient in order to understand the social, cultural, and economic nuances that might impact her health outcomes. I responded, "Priya, you're a fourth-year medical student going into adolescent psychiatry where you'll actually have the time to spend with your patients on these areas. But when we consider the absolute shortage of physicians in America, and the exaggerated shortage in Black and Mexican and poor areas of American cities, the shortage becomes oppressive, and the possibility to spend the kind of time you're talking about does not exist, then there's no reason to hope that such dedication, alone, will close the gap in health outcomes." Later, at lunch, the medical school dean said, "Man, you knew the student's name, her year in school, her specialty! I don't even know that, and I'm the dean! How did you do that?" I confessed that as people were trickling into the lecture hall, waiting for others to get their slices of free pizza, I went around and chatted with about half of the impending crowd, trying to know the audience before I was to speak.

Next, someone who can only be described as a senior professor, asked me if I'd ever considered "biological race" in my research, such as head circumference. Because I was being recorded, and YouTube was newly on the scene, I paused and allowed the professor to elongate his question as I considered what I would say—and what I would not say—in response. I noticed the uneasy expressions on the faces of Black faculty and deans in the audience, then inhaled an excessive amount of air and said, "Let me refer you to Troy Duster's book, *Backdoor to Eugenics*. I'll bet you'll find that helpful. Next question."

The Black faculty exhaled.

The Dean of Diversity came up to me after the lecture and apologized for the senior faculty member's question. I told her I'd be all right, but that I worried about his students.

I am interested in race. I read, I write, I attend lectures, I give lectures. I've always considered race as overt, up front, plain for anyone to see. I've seen postcards with pictures of lynchings where White adults and their children, with lemonade served, comprised the audience for a Black man hanging from a tree with a rope around his neck. Billie Holiday's "Strange Fruit." Race in medicine is about strokes from uncontrolled blood pressure, blindness and lower leg amputations from complications of diabetes, excess deaths.

My college roommate in the 1980s, during a late-night dorm debate, noted to the lounge of freshman when, for some odd reason, a discussion about *Happy Days* emerged, with Richie, Potsie, and Ralph enjoying their afternoons at Arnold's: "It must have been nice to be young and White in the 1950s. But they were lynching my people. Those weren't happy days for us."

It's thorny to speak about race to multiple audiences. We discuss race every day at our home, outside of our home, at every turn. White people, from what I understand, do not. A single word can make all the difference. And centuries of words about race can have no effect at all.

My family attends a Black church in our city that is a haven for Indian, Korean, Taiwanese, Chinese, and Japanese families. Two of our three children look White, which is decidedly a Mississippi reality rooted in slavery on my wife's side of the family. Our third child looks Indian, or else Oaxacan. Our children don't stand out as "minorities" in our city. Neither did my wife during her childhood in Los Angeles where she grew up with mainly other Black children, nor did I growing up in Stockton with Mexican, Filipino, Black, Japanese, and Chinese children, feel like minorities as children. She and I stand out in our new city now, however, even if our children do not. We talk about the nuances of race and hope that our children, who are not at all interested in the topic at the moment, will be a different audience, with time, and will recall these lessons with zeal in college when someone, innocently or not, asks them what they are.

I saw Rob Reiner, who played Meathead in *All in the Family,* on a flight from New Jersey. My wife and I had taken our son to visit a prestigious boarding school in the American east, as we considered sending him there for the ninth grade. Reiner boarded the plane before me, and was sitting in the aisle near the front of the plane as I made my way to the rear. I recognized him and said, "Hey. I think you're great! I saw you on TV last week and loved what you said." We mutually reached out and shook hands. Rob Reiner thanked me. By the time I reached my seat I realized that I had gotten the show wrong, but got so excited that I was actually talking about the week before when I saw him with his father, Carl Reiner, during a different interview. I wish I'd been sitting next to him so that I could correct my memory. Rob Reiner was gone by the time we landed and the back rows, where we remained, finally had the chance to exit the plane.

I sensed a stark difference between me and my son when we flew back from visiting the east coast boarding school where he was accepted. Even if I could argue that he and I are the same versions of each other separated by the decay since the 1970s, in the end, I suspect I'm wrong: My son is not a better version of me; but a magnificent version of himself.

My friend, a Wall Street investment banker, after we'd seen a play or finished an Italian dinner on the upper east side, noted about a recent economic recovery, "The economy is doing well." I clarified that this news does not affect the poor guy who can't get a job, or who is paid too little to honestly take care of his family. Then, for whom is the economy doing well? My friend and his Wall Street contemporaries, investors, share-holders, and the company leadership were represented in such a comment, but not the part-time worker without benefits, or her children, at one of those companies.

My friend smiled and pointed me to the subway. I took the stairs underground and caught the next train.

14

Bryan Stevenson

(an Epistolary Piece)

I don't remember where I heard that Yale offered a few free online courses. I couldn't be sure what this meant, but found the idea interesting. I was able to find this series on Yale's website. A few courses from previous terms had been recorded, and were available for anyone to watch. Then, it wasn't a course offering the way I understood "taking a course." Nevertheless, I looked through the list and found some that seemed interesting. I tried one, then another, and quickly didn't think I'd be interested in completing an entire semester video of a professor talking to some students in a past class. I looked through the list of course offerings one last time before I would give up.

One course caught my attention because of my own literary interests that began after I completed my formal education, so I thought I'd watch this opening class before giving up on the entire undertaking. The course was in the Spanish Department: Cervantes's *Don Quixote*. I put on my headphones, clicked on the first class, and listened for a few minutes. The professor, Roberto González Echevarría, I later found, is the world's expert on *Don Quixote*. He spent the first lecture, "Intro," discussing the book's place in world literature, the title, itself, and a few administrative class rules. I found the rhythm of the professor's speech, the profound content of even the novel's title and its pronunciation, which was a tantalizing teaser for the magnitude of what would follow in later lectures, and, above all, his sense of humor, enchanting.

I understood from his introductory remarks to the students, not to mention his status as a world thinker of the highest order, that I should not trouble him with a tiresome email, like, say, from a groupie. But since I live in California, I didn't have a way to meet him in person, if that were even possible. So, I sent him what I hoped he'd find a thoughtful email to let him know that I was a fan after only a few lectures, and that his work was already influencing my own approach to literature, and to reality.

"Dear Professor González Echevarría ...." I apologized for sending an unsolicited email, and then proceeded to tell him of my literary labyrinth that led me to the great Spaniard, Cervantes, and that I found the online course inspiring because of the particularity of González Echevarría's thinking. His response: "Thanks for your words, I am very happy to have inspired you. Do get in touch when you come to CT and we will have coffee, RGE."

I got to calling him "Roberto" in subsequent exchanges, which seemed a little uncomfortable since he'd won so many honors, was awarded the National Humanities Medal by President Obama, and wrote the Introduction to the current edition of *Don Quixote*. Our exchanges became more comfortable. We chatted as friends. I later discovered a line in his "Introduction" that I might be able to use as the epigraph to the novel I was writing: "In the fiction, as no doubt in the reader's own world, the truth is a matter of negotiation and compromise." I asked Roberto if I could use his line. He replied: "Dear Richard, you can use any line of mine for whatever purpose. We will meet soon, I am preparing courses and a lecture I have to give in Rio. Best, Roberto."

* * *

My wife and I went to see actress-playwright-professor Anna Deavere Smith speak at the public library near our house. She talked directly to the library audience, played some characters from former productions, and tried some new characters she was touching up for a future production. The present emerged right in front of us. When the talk-play ended, I wanted to meet her. There was a line of people who'd purchased books waiting for her to sign them. My wife and I bought one of the books, stood in line, and waited to get to the front where Anna Deavere Smith would sign it. We stepped closer over the next few minutes, listening to what we could hear as she talked to the others in line ahead of us. Then I was at the head of the line talking with Anna Deavere Smith. I quickly mentioned how much I enjoyed her work, and that I was inspired by her writing and acting as I was completing my own work on race and medicine.

A few days later, as I read more about her, I saw that she's a professor at NYU, and noticed her email address on the university website:

Dear Professor Smith,

My wife and I enjoyed your visit to Newport Beach Library, entirely. We were moved by your art and by your substance that, together, bespeak the urgency required to live as conscious people interested in people who appear doomed, based upon all of the evidence. When you and I briefly chatted at the library, I was so consumed by your presence that I neglected to mention that I am the adult version of the high school students from the Strawberry Mansion piece in your performance. My high school, and my childhood, were simi-

lar to what you described in the narrative in Ms. Wayman's voice. I watched the ABC video with Diane Sawyer and noted that my high school was not as dangerous. Still, I recognized the idea that children like us have so little, if anything at all, upon which to depend as we consider a life, a world, different and better than the only one we know. An impossibility save for a statistically negligible few. Still, we persist. Because of Ms. Wayman, and people like her, like you.

I became tearful as I listened to you during this part. And again, when I watched the ABC story online. Tearful because this story reminded me of my own childhood; but even more because this reality remains the present for so many.

I do what I can. Not nearly as much as you, to be sure. Thank you, again, for your work. I'm inspired, invigorated, hopeful in the face of no hope other than the tangibility of my own escape from an analogous high school experience, an analogous childhood. I won't trouble you with the details, but can say that I hope to continue my own work on race in medicine that is in keeping with your work, your leadership, your art.

I hope our paths cross again. (Certainly, I love your work on Nurse Jackie, which I watch every Sunday.) I'll be sure to let you know when my book of personal essays on health disparities is published.

In short, my wife and I were inspired and delighted. Your awesome talent and humanity help sustain us.

Sin cerely,
Richard

Dear Dr. Garcia,

Thank you for your thoughtful email. Perhaps I will have a chance to interview you in the course of developing this project.

With my best wishes,
Anna

Hey Anna,

Looking forward to seeing you in Santa Monica. My wife just got front row tickets! Again, thanks so much for your work. I'm honestly inspired by your dedication to substance with your art. I'm a fan; and trying my best to follow your lead.

Sincerely,
Richard

Bryan Stevenson (an Epistolary Piece)

Dear Anna,

We LOVED your performance last night. My wife said, "It was awesome," but meant it in the literal way, not the colloquial. We're trying to get our fourteen-year-old daughter to the show today. I don't know if I mentioned this to you before, but I am from Stockton! When you talked about the kid whose two options were prison or death, I almost cried. Those were my only options, too. Still, I went to Berkeley and medical school—like your description of the flower from the crack in the sidewalk. I was the "just one."

I'm not trying to be melodramatic here, but what you did seemed specifically for me. My new book that will be out in a few days contains chapters that consider Stockton. In fact, one of the chapters, "On Meeting Richard Rodriguez," has a scene where I say to him about leaving clinical pediatrics and becoming a writer, "But I'm from Stockton. What do I have to say?" Richard Rodriguez replied, "Everybody's from Stockton." The original title for the book was Everybody's from Stockton. The editor convinced me to change it.

Last thing: I've already written a rough draft of a chapter for my next book: "Monk Played in the Cracks." I wrote it in two sections, with a quote from D.H. Lawrence's "Poetry of the Present" initiating the first section, and a long quote from King's "Letter from Birmingham Jail" initiating the second. I referenced the "wait has almost always meant never" part. What a coincidence to hear you read the entire "Letter" onstage! I loved the accompanying music, your cadence, your crescendos. I'm so intellectually and artistically moved by your work. It's as if you're, somehow, my big sister.

The reason, entirely, that I became a pediatrician was so that I could return to Stockton to help children like me. I did that briefly, but was restless. The works of Zora Neale Hurston and Jean Toomer, Ellison, Baldwin, and the others, led me to a labyrinth of Russian and Latin American literature that brought me to my own intersection with medicine, literature, and humanity. I can only dream of following your lead now.

Sincerely, your brother,
Richard

Dear Brother Richard,

Thank you so much for this kind note. I'm very glad that the performance meant something to you.

Warm regards,
Anna

My kids' high school drama teacher knows Anna, and brought her to school to talk with the students during the day, and to the parents that evening. Anna portrayed a few character vignettes from her forthcoming show, then answered some questions from the audience of splendid parents. She eventually found her way to my side of the audience and noticed my raised hand. I can't recall my exact question, but I said something like, "Hi Anna. Your art is important. How do you see it impacting things concretely for people in need?" She listened to the end, though seemed to have the answer long before I'd finished my question. Anna said something like, "I'm an artist and a teacher. People in the audience do other things. I can only hope that my work inspires them to do their work."

* * *

I saw Bryan Stevenson, founder of the Equal Justice Initiative, in some interviews recently. Perhaps I'd seen him before. Perhaps not. The one that started things for me, where I noticed him, was when he talked about how America has never really confronted the legacy of slavery and the great evil used to legitimate slavery: the ideology of White supremacy. He went on to talk about freedom in the minds of descendants of slaves. There was a presumption of dangerousness and guilt. "I think we need truth and reconciliation in America. We've never had that."

Inspired by his enlightenment, I told my friend about Bryan Stevenson. She interrupted me because she already knew of him. In fact, her daughter, a law student, was doing an internship at the Equal Justice Initiative. I read more about Bryan Stevenson and found that his work, unlike mine, outside of clinical medicine, was concrete. His breathtaking accomplishments are both humbling and inspiring. From the Equal Justice Initiative website: "Under his leadership, EJI has won major legal challenges eliminating excessive and unfair sentencing, exonerating innocent death row prisoners, confronting abuse of the incarcerated and the mentally ill and aiding children prosecuted as adults. Mr. Stevenson has successfully argued several cases in the United States Supreme Court and recently won an historic ruling that mandatory life-without-parole sentences for all children 17 or younger are un- constitutional. Mr. Stevenson and his staff have won reversals, relief or release for over 115 wrongly condemned prisoners on death row. Mr. Stevenson has initiated major new anti-poverty and anti-discrimination efforts that challenge the legacy of racial inequality in America, including major projects to educate communities about slavery, lynching and racial segregation."

Bryan Stevenson (an Epistolary Piece)

Dear Professor Stevenson,

I saw you on TV the other night when you noted that killing a White person amounts to more than killing a Black person. I suppose I already sensed this, intuitively; but hearing that it's twenty-two times worse, in fact, concretized this sense.

I told my friend about you. She mentioned that her daughter is one of your protégés. Small world. Her mother contributed a chapter to my recent book that considers health outcomes disparities, written as personal essays with James Baldwin, Richard Rodriguez, and Montaigne in mind. These attempts rely on Aristotle's forensic discourse. We're already at work on a follow-up book that considers solutions: a critique of previously proposed solutions, and some new ideas. We are writing chapters that locate such thinking in a different context than can ordinarily be found in the medical literature. These personal essays, toward this end, will be written with Aristotle's deliberative discourse in mind.

Mainly, I just want to thank you for your stark and inspirational interview. I hope my own work addressing disparities in health out- comes between the races can be considered in keeping with your work. I don't mean to be presumptuous; rather, I'm inspired by your work. I look forward to reading and hearing more. The interview was a great interaction. Thanks for that.

Sincerely,
Richard

Dear Dr. Garcia,

Thanks so much for your email, and for letting me know about your work and writing, which sounds fantastic. I'll definitely find your book and check it out. I'm thrilled to know that you're writing about these issues, and look forward to learning more.

All the best,
Bryan

Dear Bryan,

I finally saw 13th *at a movie art house on Saturday. I was stunned by your last line. I'll have to watch it again to get that line accurately, but the sentiment is profound. It's Faulknerian: "The past isn't dead. It isn't even past." Something like that.*

I'm finishing up the final couple of chapters of my next book. I'll take the title from Fannie Lou Hamer's famous quote, "I'm sick and tired of being sick and tired." Mainly, I'm interested in framing a discussion about would-be solutions to disparities in health outcomes based on race.

A friend suggested that other possible titles, Sick and Tired: On Framing Solutions to Health Disparities

Bryan Stevenson (an Epistolary Piece)

Between Races, *or,* Monk Played in the Cracks: On Framing Solutions to Health Disparities, *might lead the reader to think that practical solutions will be forthcoming in the book. But when she read the sample chapters, she didn't find recipes that people could take and use to stamp out centuries-old disparities.*

This could be a simple thing. But it could be worse. Is it that I should not write a forensic book that considers old attempts at would-be solutions and looks to frame how future solutions might be constructed? I suppose I'm writing in the lineage of Troy Duster, Ida B. Wells's grandson, who frames how "race," itself, can be understood. (Do you know Troy?)

Your powerful last line in 13th *is paralyzing, and, at once, inspiring for people who struggle even when there's no end in sight. I'm reminded of Barbara Fields, History professor at Columbia, and her analogous comment at the end of Ken Burns' Civil War documentary. Barbara said something like, "In many ways the Civil War is still being fought. And, regrettably, it can still be lost."*

Publishing still requires double-edged discourse. I'm further inspired by what Toni Morrison said when he asked her about solutions to race. She said that White people have a serious problem. And that they should do something about it.

My friend said about my not tangibly solving the health disparities based on race: "You should not be required to solve this problem when you are not in power to solve it. The pow-

erful cannot require the victims to come up with ways to stop their oppression . . . ." (She said it better on the phone this morning.)

I understand that you're not simply writing lofty frames for people to think about; but you are actually tangibly helping people. My favorite line in Morrison's Beloved is: "This is flesh I'm talking about." I'll keep working. I'll try to come up with tangible, practical things with which to pepper my text. But I'm just a pediatrician writing personal essays when I find a few moments. Nevertheless, I read a lot, and am not able to do much on this front. So, I'll keep struggling.

In fact, I have a title for another chapter in mind: "Bryan Stevenson." With your permission, I'll write about this very struggle.

☺ Sincerely,
Richard

I decided to write to Bryan Stevenson to thank him for his work, for inspiring me to continue working toward decreasing health disparities based on race, and to confess that I think I can do more, tangible good now that I'd heard him speak. I thought about what I've done so far. More than this, I thought about what I haven't done. I remembered a phone call with a professor who'd just heard that he was declined at his university tenure review.

I, too, felt miserable about something, which I cannot now recall.

The declined professor said, "I gathered up all of my publications strewn around my messy house and stacked them into a pile. I have to admit that by the time I was finished I could see that it was an impressive pile."

When he finished chronicling his publications and lamenting his failed bid for tenure, he stopped to hear my thoughts.

I said, "There are some children alive today because of me."

My professor friend said, "You see, just to be able to say that is impressive."

But I didn't agree with him in the way he meant to compliment me. I thought that if I were not in the Emergency Room or the Pediatric ICU at those particular times, another pediatrician would have saved the babies' lives. The concrete good I did was not specific, particular to me.

In a recent talk with the great essayist, Richard Rodriguez, over dim sum in San Francisco's Chinatown, he, too, noted the impressive work I did as a pediatrician. I corrected him and said that other pediatricians could do what I do; but that if he didn't think of a thought and write it in an essay, no one else would, and the thought would not exist. I don't mean to depreciate my clinical work. But when I wonder what I might do relative to health disparities based on race that is in keeping with the corporeal concrete betterment of a baby who couldn't breathe, but now does, I'm paralyzed by the weight of the centuries. Others, too, wonder what I can do concretely, and push me for tangibility to decrease, if not eliminate, the centuries of racial oppression in my text. A wry smile.

15

Monk Played in the Cracks

I

... The poetry of the beginning and the poetry of the end must have that exquisite finality, perfection which belongs to all that is far off. It is in the realm of all that is perfect. It is of the nature of all that is complete and consummate ...

But there is another kind of poetry: the poetry of that which is at hand: the immediate present. In the immediate present there is no perfection, no consummation, nothing finished ...

Life, the ever-present, knows no finality, no finished crystallization ....

> "Poetry of the Present"
> D.H. Lawrence
> Pangbourne, 1919

We drove, passively, in a way, to find the San Francisco airport where Antoine, my friend, was to catch his plane for our senior class trip to Hawaii the summer after our high school graduation. I was not going to Hawaii, but to Berkeley from Stockton, the long way, for a summer session before my freshman year in college was to start. No money for Hawaii? Perhaps. I don't recall. But I had a job, and just as little money as Antoine, so could have gotten the money, I suppose. But I planned to attend Summer Bridge, a session at the University of California at Berkeley for minority students who were to be severely outnumbered freshman in the fall.

Because I never really left Stockton, I'd never driven across a bridge until that day. First would be the San Mateo Bridge, connecting Hayward in the east, to San Mateo, in the west; and then up the 101 North to San Francisco, and then back across the water on the Bay Bridge east to Oakland. Then, hopefully, we'd find Berkeley.

It was there, on the 101 North, either before or after we'd dropped Antoine off at SFO, on a defunct Bay Area radio station, KSOL, that I heard the chimes, the prologue, of what promised to be an eruptive song. "And I Am Telling You I'm Not Going," the reduction sauce of the Broadway musical, *Dreamgirls*, starring Jennifer Holliday. I had not yet heard Holliday's voice. I had not even heard of *Dreamgirls*, never once considered Broadway in New York as a possibility, and had no reference with which I could hear her ethos.

I don't know if my mother, Antoine, or his mother talked in the car as I drove. Sound beyond Holliday no longer existed.

It's tricky, of course, to *write* about sound. And I'd hate to be pedestrian and talk about "the quality" of Holliday's voice. This sort of thing is best done by real experts. Although, I must say, I am an expert audience member. For example, I'd already recognized Patti LaBelle's timbre, a thickness I'd discovered the year before, as her own, independent of others, without regard for, indeed, in spite of, let's say, Judy Garland. (I'd seen Patti LaBelle on TV singing "Somewhere Over the Rainbow," which I could only vaguely recognize as a song from the annual *Wizard of Oz* I'd watched on TV since before memory. LaBelle, near the end of the song, extended her arms to either side, squatted a bit, and flapped her wings as she crescendoed toward the end. "She's going to fly away," my mother cautioned.) I understood the force of Holliday's voice, a quality I'd thought of as volume until then. Though I have a dead father, a jazz trumpeter, whom I met only three or four times, I am not a musician, and had only ever lived as a jazz student. (I've considered that these two realities are genetically related, as it were.) And though the radio's volume was not turned up when I first heard Jennifer Holliday's force, I thought I'd better pay attention. Through the years, I've noticed that Holliday's timbre and power, sometimes, are replaced with a guttural call adorned with gospel grace notes and askew murmurs spaced between Holliday and the audience, inviting us, in fact, to participate.

I don't remember the sequence, but I'm certain that I heard "And I Am Telling You I'm Not Going" on the radio countless times in the freshman dorm; I bought the soundtrack, an album in those days; and later the CD; still later, I downloaded the digital versions, including the movie version with Jennifer Hudson, and the Broadway concert version, with Lillias White.

A college student in 1983, with no money of my own, I planned to see the Broadway show in San Francisco. But when the tour finally made it north from Los Angeles, I received an abdominal blow when I found that Holliday had left the tour after LA. I understood that she was to pursue her solo singing career. Nevertheless, I went to see the production with the understudy who had replaced Holliday. Because of the way the past exists—all at once—I cannot recall much about that particular show, as I've heard the recording uncountable times, and have seen many productions of the musical since that first time. (Two things stand out from that first SF show:

Arnetia Walker, at the end of "This Ain't No Party," punctuated the piece the way Holliday punctuates "And I Am Telling You I'm Not Going" with a playful, "Hey." Walker, as I recall, or imagine, showed a sly smile further noting Holliday's absence. The second thing that stands out is only circuitously relevant. In the second act, when someone asks Effie if she's going to join the lawyers as they dismantle her nemesis, former manager, and father of her daughter, Curtis, she replies, "No. I want to talk to Deena." The audience laughed at her pronunciation of "No," which was more, "Naw!" I'd forgotten who starred as Effie that first time I saw *Dreamgirls* until many years later, after I'd finished medical school and had enough wherewithal to see shows on Broadway, I sat in the back of the orchestra section of *The Life* in 1997 and heard one of the leading characters, an aged, languid prostitute, say, "Naw!" I instantly turned to my wife and whispered, "That's her! Lillias White. I saw her in San Francisco in 1983!" My wife said, "You mean from 'Naw' you went all the way back?"

I smiled. Satisfied.

I've thought about this story intermittently for thirty-seven years since that first time I heard Jennifer Holliday's voice on the freeway. The totality of the story emerged for me gradually, and then all at once. A friend mentioned this emergence to me in a different context when I was complaining about something I've forgotten about by now. He said that as a *conscious* person it was difficult for me to accept whatever it was I was complaining about. I completely agreed with him, noted his point of view, and went on to think of myself as a conscious person from that moment forward. I've even used this imperceptible example in discussions with other people. That is, if I'm "conscious" now, it began on the way to Berkeley. Hearing that song—and, more importantly, being conscious of hearing that song, which is different, entirely, from my passively hearing everything else before—marks the beginning of an onomatopoeic version of my becoming conscious.

My wife and I went to see Jennifer Holliday's concert at the Cerritos Center a few years ago. We stayed after the show to meet her. (I think we saw Cheryl Lynn in the audience!) Nervous, I stood in a line of people who waited backstage. Jennifer Holliday emerged and greeted us, each one, with a few words and a hug. When she approached me, I lost all of my good sense, and said, "I'm a pediatrician, and I left my patients behind to see you." Or something like that. But this wasn't true. I had the night off. I simply had so much to say, had lost my wits, and this was all I could say, evidently. I wanted to tell her about hearing her for the first time that summer after high school . . . .

She laughed and gave me a hug.

Still, I had never seen Jennifer Holliday in *Dreamgirls*. I read that she would be starring in an Atlanta production a few years ago, so we flew there to see her. Since we'd never been to Atlanta, we made it a long weekend. Indeed, we went to the theater the night before our scheduled show and found that we could get tickets for that night, too. "We can see her twice!"

I watched a YouTube video of Paul Simon's "Bridge Over Troubled Water." Paul Simon, whom I like, started. Then Jennifer Holliday joined him. Naturally, she delivered a powerful, gospel redirection which invited me to pay attention the *way* I paid attention to her gospel version of "Short People" when she guest starred on an *Ally McBeal* episode during its first season on TV. (I bought the entire series and can listen to Jennifer Holliday in her choir robe anytime I want: "They got, uh, little voices going peep, peep, peep.") Luther Vandross joined them next and redirected the Simon song again toward Vandross's style, per se, which isn't all that far from gospel, though not quite as proximate as Holliday's. Quickly, Vandross and Holliday entered into a call and response that included me, I admit, as a virtual audience responding to the calls. Vandross escalated the dialogue in a challenge, it seemed, to which Holliday lifted her left hand and hollered a rhythmic retort that, in turn, inspired Vandross, and let him know that she was not going away. Paul Simon seemed to understand that he should stay out of this vociferous discourse, more moaning and hollering than singing, assured that he'd penned a great song worthy of such majestic hollering.

From that first time on the 101 North through now, I wonder how I can make sense of Jennifer Holliday. Her matriculation through art. What *she* means, and can mean, to a voice that lands upon an audience. Of my own role as audience to her character onstage. That is, what audience am I? Becoming "conscious," it seems, landed me squarely in the present.

I didn't see Sarah Vaughan. Had not yet become a fan of jazz when I was at Berkeley. I did note that she was to play the Greek Theater on Berkeley's campus. I didn't go to see her. Years later, after I'd become a jazz fan, in general, and a Sarah Vaughan fan, in particular, I planned to see her at the Greek Theater in Los Angeles. I believe this performance was cancelled. Sarah Vaughan died a little later. I listen to her live recordings and cannot understand why I didn't see her at the Berkeley Greek. Or what took me so long to become a jazz fan. I imagine a movie about Sarah Vaughan titled *Sassy* or *The Devine One* or *Once in a*

While. The first scene opens with a laminar flow of smoke rising from a cigarette upward until the smoke becomes turbulent flow. Pan out. She's sitting at a nightclub after the show talking to the guys. Starring Alfre Woodard. Joe Williams is there. (Starring Jamie Foxx?)

Angela Bofill had a stroke. She's getting better, I hear. We saw her in Las Vegas once. The crowd was sparse. The club, The Blue Note—Las Vegas, is now an all-you-can-eat sushi restaurant. (I've never been.) Bofill played the timbales and sang her 80s R&B with a Latin take. New Yorican. Cuban. Black. The crowd was small—about twelve of us, I'm sure. I could not distinguish how the show might have been different had the place been crowded with a big audience. Neither could she, she told us between songs. "I'm on Your Side," a song that Jennifer Holliday, coincidently, had already remade.

I saw Rachelle Ferrell a few times around Los Angeles. The first was in Redondo Beach at a defunct nightclub, The Strand, which is now a Bristol Farms Market. Will Downing walked up out of the audience onto the stage to sing their duet, "Nothing Has Ever Felt Like This." Then three or four more times in Hollywood. At the piano, she sang to us in the audience, and to the others onstage. She listened, too, to her band members onstage, and to us, in the audience. In an unrelated episode, as we connected flights from somewhere to home in LA, my wife saw her at an airport. "Look!" my wife said to me. In a panic, I introduced myself to Rachelle Ferrell and told her that we'd seen her many times. I mentioned the Will Downing duet at The Strand. Ferrell smiled and said, "That was a long time ago." Delighted, I said, "I'll see you in LA next time." [Hey Rachelle!]

Ralph Ellison teaches us in his *Invisible Man* that the past is prologue. While I'm not prepared for a metaphysical collaborative with Ellison, the past can also be past, unscrutinized, if I'm not careful. That is to say, I hear there's a musician on the scene. Esperanza Spalding. I have not yet heard any of her music. I have not seen her. But I understand that she'll be playing nearby soon. Jason Moran, too, is on the scene. Inspired by Monk, whom I didn't hear until late. We saw Moran in San Francisco for the first time at the new SF Jazz Center. While I cannot put into words what we heard, even as Moran played some spoken words into his piano, I considered that jazz is a *way* to think. I'm a more deliberate audience now. No more passive listening. But alive.

II

> ... We know through painful experience that freedom is never voluntarily given by the oppressor; it must be demanded by the oppressed. Frankly, I have yet to engage in a direct action campaign that was "well timed" in the view of those who have not suffered unduly from the disease of segregation. For years now I have heard the word "Wait!" It rings in the ear of every Negro with piercing familiarity. This "Wait" has almost always meant "Never."
>
> ... There comes a time when the cup of endurance runs over, and men are no longer willing to be plunged into the abyss of despair. I hope, sirs, you can understand our legitimate and unavoidable impatience....
>
> "Letter from Birmingham Jail"
> The Reverend Dr. Martin Luther King, Jr.
> Birmingham, 1963

My best man, Mark White, a professor of classical rhetoric, taught King's "Letter from Birmingham Jail" in his classes through the years. While Mark was never my professor, I was most certainly his student. I asked him about King's argument against waiting, thinking that Mark would take off on one of his insightful lessons about race. I thought he would continue in the same vein as King and further explain the urgency. But Mark surprised me with his answer. He pointed out the flaw in King's argument: "We've waited this long. What's a couple more weeks?"

Mark argued that it's not the *amount of time* that's at issue; but the very content of King's examples. Pointing to the duration was a more palatable argument for the intended audience (both the clergy and the rest of America) than pointing to the inhumanity when trying to appeal to an audience invested in continued delay.

Then, the *reason* for the urgency to reach equality was not going to be best described in moral terms, but in temporal ones, when considering the audience. I am only a few months younger than King's "Letter," and have learned throughout my life that a moral argument can reach a peak, then slide back down its Sisyphean slope.

I am a doctor. I chose medicine for the standard reasons minorities choose medicine: as a social and personal place in the world that rejects the past, along with its future arc, in favor of the present. The urgent present. Now, where the past is upon us in its fullness, tantalizing us in medicine as we reconcile science and humanity, history and the personal pronoun, I.

The chronicle of inequalities in health between the races is captured in hundreds of medical articles as described in the 2002 Institute of Medicine Report, *Unequal Treatment*. So-called social determinants are implicated, along with overt racism, generational wealth disparities, unequal geographic access to doctors, and the like.

But what can anyone *do* about these so-called social determinants?

In his 1964 State of the Union Address, President Lyndon B. Johnson said, "Unfortunately, many Americans live on the outskirts of hope—some because of their poverty, and some because of their color, and all too many because of both. Our task is to help replace their despair with opportunity. This administration today, here and now, declares unconditional war on poverty in America . . . ." There was no War on Color. (Or was there?) I suppose that war has been ongoing. The War on Poverty is unwinnable. From antiquity until now, and beyond, it's unwinnable en masse in our society. Then why write an essay? A book? Which book has changed things for the better with respect to race? What troubles me about writing, it's blasphemous for me to say here, I understand, is what comes from the Mexican poet, Octavio Paz, in his essay "Quantity and Quality," where he teaches us: "The past and future vanish, and the present intensifies into a single instant: the three times are exhaled in one breath. The instant explodes and dissipates."

But what collection of words will help us arrive at a better present where race and medicine collide, still, in our history? What collection of sentences can we use to direct our efforts to treat this past, this present? Who is this "we"? And what can we do?

In his 1966 speech "The Rhetorical Situation," Lloyd F. Bitzer said:

> " . . . a work of rhetoric is pragmatic; it comes into existence for the sake of something beyond itself; it functions ultimately to produce action or change in the world; it performs some task. In short, rhetoric is a mode of altering reality, not by the direct application of energy to objects, but by the creation of discourse which changes reality through the mediation of thought and action. The rhetor alters reality by bringing into existence a discourse of such a character that the audience, in thought and action, is so engaged that it becomes mediator of change. In this sense rhetoric is always persuasive . . . . Prior to the creation and presentation of discourse, there are three constituents of any rhetorical situation: the first is the *exigence* . . . Any *exigence* is an imperfection marked

by urgency; it is a defect, an obstacle, something waiting to be done . . . Finally, rhetorical situations come into existence, then either mature and decay or mature and persist . . ."

What is the exigency relevant to disparities in health based on race today if we can codify these disparities back to at least our Civil War? Why now? Is it King's caution that because the disparities have persisted for so long, then it's about time? Or is it about something other than time? Time as a variable, if we can conceive of time in this way, stretching from before time to after time, right through now. Now is where the Mexican diabetic woman finds herself. The Black woman with cancer. The Black baby born too soon who struggles mightily, in her tiny form, before she dies.

I sometimes think about my dead childhood friends and wonder what, if anything, could have saved them: one dead in a crack deal, another from a stroke, I think, and another from complications of diabetes. All desperately young; all dead like soldiers of the past and of the future.

I also sometimes think that I could have died along with them. This has always been the rub of my own condition as a doctor. I examined the possibilities of my adolescence and understood that I was meant for some other world. I don't mean that colloquially, but like August Wilson meant it in *Joe Turner's Come and Gone* when Herald Loomis said in the dénouement, ". . . so I can get my a starting place in the world. The world got to start somewhere. That's what I been looking for. I been wandering a long time in somebody else's world . . . I can say my goodbye and make my own world."

The null hypothesis for children in my family for all of the generations leading up to me, from either side, was that we were all doomed. I lived with this, passively, in a way, even as I went to college and medical school; into clinical practice and executive medicine; throughout medicine and into writing personal essays, fiction, and drama. I never questioned the negligible differences between me and what could have happened to me growing up in that place where some of us don't live to adulthood, or don't live free in adulthood, or don't have much of a life to live, at all, en route to early and miserable deaths.

I rejected the null hypothesis in spite of all versions of reality available to me.

On a weekend home from college before heading to medical school, out with my friends at a club or a parking lot, one of them, proud of me in all respects, asked, "How old will you be when you're a doctor?"

I said, "Twenty-six." I paused, and then said, "You'll be twenty-six, too, when I'm a doctor."

There exists a complicated interdisciplinarity in my own approach to life and medicine that is a weight for me. Science, math, literature, medicine, social science, music. I'm cognizant that a medical audience might be disinterested in synecdoche or metonymy. That I might best serve people by diagnosing something early, treating them correctly, imparting healthy advice. I am inspired, however, by what appears to be a required complicated approach to addressing health disparities insofar as practical solutions, resulting in concrete betterment, reside in an inextricably intertwined gospel call and response with a complicated audience.

I watched an interview with a tenth-grade student in London who invented an app that can summarize an article into an abstract, which is good for someone in a hurry, someone in line getting coffee with only enough time to read a summary of an article. A virtual *CliffsNotes* of yore. Then, should the hurried, caffeinated reader be interested in the full article, based on its virtual abstract, she could read more later. The young Londoner was coy, but seems to have sold this app for thirty million dollars, give or take. I couldn't help but wonder about the content, itself, independent of the abstract. This depth, it would appear, is not worth nearly as much. What remains most valuable, by all accounts, is the superficial summary of content written by some other, real, cheaper writer.

Sick and Tired

I have a premium cable TV package that gets more than nine hundred channels. I only watch about ten of them. Maybe more. As I did something (I don't remember now), one of the music channels played in the background. Channel nine hundred thirty something, as I recall. I was not actively listening, but did note a very nice drum solo during one of the pieces. I stopped, looked at the TV, noted the piece, and decided I'd buy it when I had the chance. I went back to doing something and noticed another great solo—saxophone this time—about twenty minutes later. I looked up to see who *this* was so that I could add this piece, too, to my burgeoning jazz collection. It was the same piece! Coltrane. *A Love Supreme.* I was a little ashamed of myself for not knowing it already.

I watched a Thelonious Monk documentary and listened to him talk. And to people talk about him. One of the discussants said about Monk during his nights as the house pianist in 1940s Minton's Playhouse on 118th: I knew guys who played the white keys, and I knew guys who played the black keys. Monk played in the cracks.

Jason Moran, inspired by Monk, played Fats Waller in San Francisco Thursday night. Moran, who played alone in San Francisco, took a break and walked back stage while some music, or voice narrative of Adrian Piper, perhaps, played overhead. Moran returned to the piano wearing an enormous mask of Fats Waller smiling, a cigarette hanging obliquely from his virtual mouth. Fats Waller turned to the audience and smiled at us as he played.

Jazz is a *way* to think, to evaluate race and its contentious, entangled world. Jazz can also be a *way* to negotiate what we'll do in medicine when race conflates our understanding of what's possible. That is, here, in the cracks, is where we find ourselves as we consider what can be done in the face of centuries of race that promise never to end; where a scientific or political or social or financial discourse works to close the gap in health outcomes between the races; where some of the proposed solutions are flaccid while unproposed ones are unheard, or not yet created. Conscious. The cracks. Terra incognita. The present.

www.ingramcontent.com/pod-product-compliance
Lightning Source LLC
Chambersburg PA
CBHW021059080526
44587CB00010B/310